Cameral Analysis

Cameral Analysis offers a theoretical explanation of the hypnotic phenomenon in neuropsychological terms and an analytical method of treating the neuroses derived from this theory.

Considering the origin of the neuroses to lie in the different methods of the two hemispheres in processing the same information, David Pedersen clearly outlines his treatment method. This is designed to expose the presence of any such information-processing discrepancies by separately analysing the verbal, non-emotional left hemisphere in the normal conscious state, and the non-verbal, emotional right hemisphere under hypnosis. This separate chamber (cameral) technique then goes on to conciliate the two hemispheres by a variety of methods.

In offering a practical non-drug treatment of psychoneuroses through hypnosis, *Cameral Analysis* will be of considerable interest to all psychotherapists, general practitioners and clinical psychologists.

David Pedersen has had 35 years' experience of the use of hypnosis in general and private practice and has written and lectured extensively on the subject. He is a past President of the Section of Hypnosis and Psychosomatic Medicine of the Royal Society of Medicine, and is a member of many other related professional bodies throughout the world.

Cameral Analysis

A Method of Treating the Psychoneuroses Using Hypnosis

David L. Pedersen

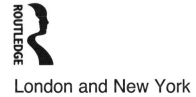

London and New York

First published 1994
by Routledge
11 New Fetter Lane, London EC4P 4EE

Simultaneously published in the USA and Canada by Routledge
29 West 35th Street, New York, NY 10001

© 1994 David L. Pedersen

Typeset in Times by Florencetype, Kewstoke, Avon
Printed and bound in Great Britain by
Biddles Ltd, Guildford and King's Lynn

British Library Cataloguing in Publication Data
A catalogue record for this book is available from the British Library

Library of Congress Cataloging in Publication Data
Pedersen, David L. (David Lawrence), 1925–
  Cameral analysis: a method of treating the psychoneuroses
using hypnosis / David L. Pedersen.
    p.   cm.
    Includes bibliographical references and indexes.
  1. Neuroses – Treatment. 2. Hypnotism – Therapeutic use.
  3. Cerebral dominance. I. Title. [DNLM: 1. Hypnosis. 2. Neurotic
Disorders – therapy. 3. Dominance, Cerebral. WM 415 P371c 1994]
RC530.P43 1994
616.89′162 – dc20
DNLM/DLC
for Library of Congress   93–37852
                                                                   CIP

ISBN 0–415–10424–6 (hbk)
ISBN 0–415–10425–4 (pbk)

Dedicated to my family, from grandparents to grandchildren

Contents

Figures

Foreword

Richard Tilleard-Cole

This scholarly work of Dr Pedersen makes for compulsive reading. In it he reveals how his concept of cameral analysis may be undertaken for the treatment of the neuroses, utilizing the specialized technique of hypnosis. He illustrates the successful working of this technique by a fascinating series of case histories. Among these the case of Mrs X and its remarkable outcome gives food for very deep thought and illustrates the advanced skill that Dr Pedersen brings to bear upon his patients. The role of the right cerebral hemisphere is seen by Dr Pedersen as being fundamental in the prevailing state of hypnosis. Its role furthermore is stressed in the production and appreciation of both music and poetry, where the author's emphasis on the bicameral route is again profoundly interesting and absorbing.

Dr Pedersen's earlier interest in the disciplines of both neurology and psychiatry place him in a most advantageous position to explore the controversial division of the human mind into the contrasting yet basic functions of the left cerebral hemisphere subserving the process of logic, and the right cerebral hemisphere subserving the process of emotion. In attributing the role of the right hemisphere in the hypnotic state, abreaction is considered to form an integral part of the treatment based on cameral analysis.

These engaging theories, with supporting experimental outcome, must, however, be taken carefully and seen to constitute what is a most impressive hypothesis. The tenets of Gestalt psychology can never be more applicable than when dealing with total cerebral function. Such concepts as perception, creative ability, the recording of experience, aptitude and the manifold ingredients of personality will always be explained in terms of concerted cerebral activity as a 'whole' and any reduction of such complicated neural function is in danger of producing its own hazards.

Yet this in no way detracts from Dr Pedersen's concepts. His patients have found the greatest help in his application of cameral analysis, and, in fact, he has succeeded where others failed.

His acknowledged professionalism as a clinician – no less than as an expert in the field of hypnosis – is most clearly supported by his text. His place is among the leaders of bicameral theory, and he stands an undisputed authority in the practice of cameral analysis by hypnosis.

R.R. Tilleard-Cole MA, BM, BCh, FRCPsych, DPM
Professor of Psychiatry, Worcester College, Oxford, and
President, Oxford Institute of Psychiatry

Foreword

Dabney M. Ewin

A new way of conceptualizing hypnosis arrived with Roger Sperry's elucidation of how the right brain thinks. From Mesmer to the present day, the story of hypnosis has been one of many observations of phenomena, with little agreement on theory. There is a similarity with diabetes. Diabetes textbooks early in this century were multi-volume tomes of observations and theories resembling the *Encyclopaedia Britannica*. Since the discovery of insulin, a 300-page text can amply supply the physician's needs for understanding and treating diabetes.

For the clinician, Sperry's Nobel Prize-winning studies on patients whose hemispheres had been surgically divided finally makes some sense of all those observations and 'laws'. In practice, it is easy to picture trance as a shift into dreamy, drive-dominated, non-verbal right brain-type thinking, while logical and verbal left brain-type thinking is simply normal waking consciousness. Freud recognized two types of thinking: primary process, 'an alogical, drive-dominated process whose influence is best seen in dreams and slips of the tongue'; and secondary process, in which 'logical, reality-bound considerations determine the association between ideas'. Since Freud was familiar with hypnosis, it is odd that he did not identify primary process with 'trance logic', though he did recognize its primacy.

Hypnotists generally accept the law of dominant effect, which states that when the will and imagination are at odds, the imagination tends to win. Based on Sperry's studies, one can substitute left brain for will, and right brain for imagination, and observe that when the two are at odds, the right brain will dominate. This is readily seen in the phobic person whose logical left brain says it is safe in the elevator, but whose right brain imagines disaster – the imagination wins and he climbs up five floors. The law of reversed effect says that if a person fears he cannot do something, the harder he *tries* the more likely he is to fail. To *try* is the most logical (left brain thinking) thing one can do, but the problem is in the emotional right brain. I only use the word 'try' when I don't want something to happen. Picture the difference between having your dentist say 'Try to relax' and just saying 'Relax'.

All this makes it imperative for the clinician to find a way to access the right brain, and Pedersen believes that that is what occurs in hypnosis. In 1984 he said:

> A subject in an hypnotic state is functioning in a uni-cameral mode, namely that of the right hemisphere. At the same time the verbal function of the subject's left hemisphere, normally available for reference, has been substituted for that of the hypnotist.

Since the verbal left brain is often shut down during highly emotional incidents (spontaneous trance or dissociation), it is understandable that the patient's conscious history often omits the incident and gives only its 'logical' rationalization of the problem. This is nicely illustrated in the fascinating case of Mrs X in this book. Her waking history gives little insight into the real origin of her panic attacks, and it is only in trance that the emotionally blocked information and remarkable solution pour out. She did not wish to be treated with drugs, and it is doubtful that she would have recovered without the cameral (hypnotic) analysis.

Our patients are not split-brained, and have functioning hemispheres on both sides that interact continuously, even in deep trance as shown by PET (positron emission tomography) scans and EEG (electroencephalography). The right hemisphere shows some increase in certain EEG waves during deep trance, but not enough to perceive trance as an *anatomical* shift. I conceive it as a shift in *type of thinking* from secondary to primary process, or in light of Sperry's work, a shift into right brain-type information processing. Certainly the many phenomena of the ordinary hypnotic trance are typical of the thought-processes of the right brain.

Dabney M. Ewin, MD, FACS
President, American Society of Clinical Hypnosis

Preface

The objectives in my writing this book are twofold: firstly, to offer a theoretical explanation of the hypnotic phenomenon in neuro-anatomical and psychophysiological terms; and secondly, to introduce an analytical method of treating the neuroses developed from such a neuropsychological theory.

The model of brain-function I use for these purposes is a hybrid of Paul MacLean's 'triune brain' theory[1] and Roger Sperry's concept of 'two separate conscious entities in one bony cranium', developed from his work on the functional lateralization of the brain's two cerebral hemispheres.[2,3,4]

MacLean has shown that any stimulus originating externally or internally, objectively or subjectively, is progressively influenced by the brain's three evolutionary formations to reach a behavioural conclusion. Sadly, this conclusion, he maintains, is never a purely logical one because of the subjective influence of genetic material from the individual's ancestral past, in particular the emotional interpretation provided by the limbic system (MacLean's paleomammalian formation). Furthermore, from MacLean's work on psychomotor epilepsy there is evidence that the limbic system supplies the neural substrate of, among other things, the sense of conviction as to what is false or true. This raises the possibility that the belief of truth or falsity depends on a primitive brain lacking in verbal comprehension and has prompted MacLean to raise the following question:

> It is one thing to have a primitive, illiterate mind for judging the authenticity of food or a mate, but where do we stand if we must depend on that same mind for belief in our ideas, concepts and theories?

Another outcome of MacLean's research is evidence that logic and emotion are the product of different cerebral mechanisms, and he concludes that this dichotomy could give the brain the capability, in certain abnormal circumstances, to dissociate into emotional and intellectual mentation.

This is similar indeed to Freud's conception of 'primary process' and 'secondary process' thinking; another comparison can be drawn with Sperry's left brain- and right brain-type of information processing. Ewin quite rightly points out in his Foreword to this book that an individual in an hypnotic state exhibits many of the illogical and emotional features characteristic of primary process thinking and right brain information processing. As a result, he prefers to relate the hypnotic state as a shift in type of thinking rather than an anatomical transfer of dominance to the right hemisphere. If we differ at all it is only to a very minor degree. Why I prefer to include the concept of an anatomical shift is because I believe that an individual in an hypnotic state not only thinks in the spatially synthetic terms typical of right hemisphere processing but can be shown to exhibit the skills of that hemisphere which we know are anatomically contained therein.

Although the origin of *emotional behaviour* can be shown to emanate from the limbic system, it is only expressible through the neocortex (MacLean's neomammalian brain) and as such must be influenced and modified by this organ. Similarly, any primitive *intellectual or logical behaviour* would evolve and also find expression through the neocortex. In the evolution of logical behaviour the main advances would have to be in the development of a highly sophisticated communication system. It would appear that in humans the neomammalian brain has taken the primitive audio-vocal communication system of the paleomammalian brain and from it developed a lexicon of sounds we recognize as speech.

In the light of Sperry's work, this giant evolutionary leap, placing humans, as it does, at the head of the mammalian evolutionary chain, seems to have necessitated a degree of anatomical separation of the logical and emotional elements of behaviour into the left and right neocortices (hemispheres). In making this division Nature has raised the possibility of purely logical thought unencumbered by the illogicality of emotion.

I am aware that this model of brain-function is relatively uncomplicated and many may consider it too simple and speculative. All I can say in defence of its simplicity is that Nature has often been found to work this way as in, for instance, the double helix structure of DNA. With regard to its speculative nature, anyone who has witnessed the quite extraordinary phenomenon of the hypnotic state cannot fail to be fascinated and intrigued both by its origin and implications. For instance, a demonstration of the return of speech under hypnosis in a patient with an hysterical paralysis of the vocal cords, or the operative removal of a uterus without the use of an anaesthetic, is bound to raise neurological questions and stimulate research in this aspect of the subject. To me, the neuropsychological model, rather than a purely psychological model, not only offers a more satisfactory route to the explanation of such an altered state of consciousness, but in doing so has stimulated the development of a treatment method that can be seen to work. It is my hope that others will be encouraged to consider, take up, add to, develop and further refine cameral analysis as a safe and effective weapon in the fight against the neuroses.

Acknowledgements

The late Dr Gordon Ambrose, some years ago, insisted that at some point I should make the time to publish my material on hypnosis. As he was one of the leading figures in the United Kingdom on the subject, I took his insistence as a compliment and promised him I would give it careful thought. This book is the result and I would like to record my thanks for the forceful part he played in its conception.

Most of the theoretical material in this volume has already appeared in papers I have given at courses, congresses or society meetings. Some of these papers have been published subsequently, and I am indebted to the editors of the *Journal of the Royal Society of Medicine*, the *Journal of the European Society of Hypnosis and Psychosomatic Medicine*, and the *Journal of the American Society of Clinical Hypnosis* for permission to use the material freely in its present form and context.

My thanks are also due to the following publishers and authors for their permission for me to use and quote from their work: Butterworth-Heinemann Ltd, for the use of 4 illustrations and text from *An Approach to Neuroanatomical and Neurochemical Psychophysiology* by L. Valzelli (1980); The Plenum Publishing Corporation for figures and text from *The Integrated Mind* by M.S. Gazzaniga and J.E. Le Doux (1978); Oxford University Press for figures and text from a paper by Jerre Levy and Colin Trevarthen appearing in *Brain*, vol. 100 (1977), pp. 105–118; The Reproductions Office of the National Gallery, London, for supplying a print of Botticelli's *Venus and Mars*; Macmillan Academic and Professional Ltd for an extensive quotation from T.R. Blakeslee's book *The Right Brain* (1980).

I would like to express my thanks to the many colleagues and friends for their support and encouragement in the preparation of this book; in particular, to the helpful discussions with psychiatrists Dr Godfrey Briggs, Dr John Farley, Dr Sarah Pedersen and Dr Peter Mellett, as well as general practitioners Dr Colin Wright and the late Dr Martin Thomas.

I am especially grateful to Professor Richard Tilleard-Cole and Dr Dabney Ewin for contributing the Forewords, which I much appreciate.

Finally, my thanks to the Bodleian Library, Oxford, and the Library of the Royal Society of Medicine, London, for the facilities offered and for the courtesy and efficiency of their staff.

Introduction

My introduction to hypnosis was as a pre-clinical student in Cambridge in 1945. A lecture, given in the physiology laboratory by Dr Bannister of the Cambridge Department of Psychology on the subject of 'suggestion', ended by his giving a demonstration of hypnosis on a volunteer from the student audience. I think the majority of those present enjoyed the lecture in the sense that it was entertaining and certainly different from the usual run of the mill, but to me it was more than impressive. By an extraordinary coincidence I had been bludgeoned into reading a biography of Sigmund Freud at the insistence of a fellow student in my digs. In this book it was stated that Freud's discovery of the unconscious mind came about after he had questioned a patient of Dr Liébault's in the latter's clinic in Nancy. Under hypnosis this patient had been given a post-hypnotic suggestion that in the waking state she would perform a certain task but would have no knowledge as to why she had performed this task. Freud was able to question her afterwards and was satisfied that she indeed had no knowledge of why she had carried out this task. From this Freud deduced that there was part of her mind which was inaccessible to her in her waking state and therefore unconscious.

All this was fresh in my mind, but before this lecture I had never witnessed this so-called 'hypnotic state' nor the method by which it was induced. It fascinated me and was the start of my lifelong interest in the subject.

It seems strange to me now to think that had I not read the biography of Freud I might never have entertained the subject of hypnosis again. I must explain how a simple thing like an argumentative discussion on human behaviour in Tulliver's coffee-house in

Cambridge all those years ago has led to me write this book. To do this I must go back to 1944 and a hardly recognizable, much camouflaged university.

It is an interesting piece of history to record that the Medical College of St Bartholomew's Hospital – the ancient mother hospital of the Empire – had suffered severely in the Blitz, which devastated the whole of the City of London surrounding St Paul's Cathedral in the early years of the war. The bombs not only blew the masonary apart but also had the effect of scattering the human infrastructure all over the Home Counties and even further afield. And so it came about that the entire pre-clinical staff and student body found themselves evacuated to Cambridge in 1941, where they remained ensconced in the greater part of Queens' College for the 'duration'.

We, as evacuees, found ourselves in a very privileged position in this great city. We enjoyed all the facilities of the Cambridge University medical faculty along with its student amenities, as well as the quietude of the 'backs' and the riotude of the 'rags' which coloured varsity living. At the same time we had the added good fortune, as Bart's students, not to come under the restrictive jurisdiction of the Cambridge University proctors. To my knowledge we never abused this freedom, and I think, in a small way, we helped that ancient institution to take a fresh look at some of its more outdated regulations, which later resulted in their post-war abolition.

In those pre-clinical years in Cambridge there were never enough rooms in Queens' College to house all its students. As a result, everyone at some point was hived off into digs licensed by the college. I found myself, along with two other Bart's students and a Portuguese postgraduate, allocated rooms at 9 DeFreville Avenue. The landlady who ran this establishment was a seventy-year-old widow who looked like a pantomime witch. She was about 5 foot 2 and bent almost double, always wore the same clothes – a brown skirt and a faded pink, woolly cardigan – and pottered about talking to herself, frequently cackling at some cloistered joke. The only food she provided was breakfast, which was really just as well when we learnt, a few days after our arrival, that in 1936 her second husband had committed suicide by gassing himself in the very oven she still used for cooking!

I never really enjoyed breakfast in those digs. George Alacao, the Portuguese postgraduate, used to pour tea over his cornflakes and slurp up the hot mixture like a bowl of soup; he drank the cold milk separately!

Kingsley Jones, an earnest Bart's student from Pontypridd and an early riser, often regaled the breakfast room with quotes from the *Daily Worker*, a communist newspaper. Jones never addressed anyone in particular, just the room. Answering comments were few unless John Farley was present, and this only occurred if it happened to be one of those very rare occasions when Farley actually got up for breakfast! The conversation was always brief and rarely extended beyond 'Shut up!'

It was Farley who lent me the biography of Freud after a fierce argument which ended by his insisting that I become acquainted with Freudian theory before attempting to converse with him again on the subject.

John Farley was the third Bart's student in the digs, and knew exactly where he was going. After qualifying he would immediately specialize in psychiatry. He had two all-engrossing passions in his life: one was the internal combustion engine, in the shape of powerful motorcycles and racing cars; the other was to understand human behaviour. He possessed an immense knowledge of both subjects. He was in the process of designing and building a sprint racing car, at the same time he had acquired (and was continually adding to) a substantial library of books on psychological theory, from Havelock Ellis through psychoanalysis to the latest Jungian and Adlerian theories. He duly specialized in psychiatry, and in the mid-1970s published a genetic theory of schizophrenia.[1]

Farley showed that there was experimental evidence that much of human social behaviour is learnt on the basis of innate neurophysiological mechanisms. He suggested that the genetic predisposition to schizophrenia consists of a deficiency in those innate mechanisms involved in acquiring non-verbal communication, imitation and language. A child so endowed would have great difficulty relating to, and empathizing with, his mother and his family, and would tend to mature into a socially inept, withdrawn and schizoid personality, vulnerable to schizophrenia if put under social pressure. Recently, a considerable body of experimental evidence has been accumulating which supports the theory, and Farley is currently busy preparing a general review of these data.

Farley's enthusiasm for the psychosomatic approach to medicine rubbed off on all his student friends and acquaintances, and I hold him, and his personal library, entirely responsible for the knowledge I had on this subject when, as a clinical student, I began to relate hypnosis to the treatment of neuroses. I owe him this debt.

After witnessing the demonstration of hypnosis I began reading more about the subject. I bought a second-hand book (which I still have to this day) from David's Bookshop just off the Market Square in Cambridge: *Methods and Uses of Hypnosis and Self-Hypnosis*. It was written by Bernard Hollander, who was a doctor practising at 57 Wimpole Street in the 1920s and 1930s. The book was first published in 1928 but my cheap edition was reprinted in 1935. David's Bookshop had priced the second-hand copy at 5 shillings, quite expensive for an impecunious student, but as all students knew, second-hand prices could be subject to negotiation and I eventually walked away with a smile, the book and a receipt for 3 shillings. I was not to know at the time, but this 3 bobs' worth was to influence my medical thinking almost as much as an expensive textbook of medicine.

Although Hollander's book is very short (only 190 pages), it is comprehensive enough to convey a very good idea of hypnosis (and its therapeutic application) in a simple and direct way most useful to a student. A great deal of its content is as relevant today as when it was first written. It stimulated me at that time to 'experiment' on my friends in Cambridge and later, as a clinical student at Bart's (then back in London), I was able to observe its use in the Psychiatric Department under the direction of its chief, Dr E.B. Strauss.

Dr Strauss was probably one of the very few psychiatrists in England who was actively interested at that time in the hypnotic phenomenon. He had written a lengthy chapter on hypnosis in a British textbook of psychiatry but, for a variety of reasons, he rarely mentioned it in teaching sessions. In the first instance, his department had been the most widely scattered of all during the war, ranging from Friern Barnet to St Albans, which effectively cut down the number and content of his lectures. In addition, clinical students approaching their final examinations knew that there was only one question on psychiatry in the whole of the papers, and what is more, this was included in the 'choice' section and was not compulsory!

Finally, there was no doubt that psychiatry in those days was considered a postgraduate subject and the teaching of it was practically ignored by the majority of medical and surgical consultants attached to the college. This is not to suggest that it was considered unimportant but rather that it took up students' time which was better spent on more basic training. It was a great compliment to Dr Strauss and the way that he conducted his out-patient teaching sessions that, under these circumstances, he was able to attract students in the numbers he did.

I enjoyed my attachment to his department. I think Dr Strauss was surprised to find among his few clinical students someone who had quite a detailed knowledge of hypnosis and was well acquainted with Freudian, Jungian and other aspects of psychological theory. He assumed I would take up psychiatry as a postgraduate subject and gave me every encouragement to learn more about it by allowing me to 'sit in', as a quiet observer, on outpatient treatments usually confined to postgraduate students. As there were very few of the latter there was never any problem involved, and it was in this way that I came to witness many cases of shell-shock treated by the abreaction of the initiating extremes of stress.

Witnessing abreaction as I did in these shell-shocked patients had a profound effect on me. Seeing a patient ducking from bullets, shouting orders, screaming oaths, fighting a hand-to-hand battle was astounding enough in itself, but to know that the patient was not an actor merely playing a part but that I was seeing a real, live performance once staged in some remote French village in the wartime theatre of operations was quite incredible. Add to this the frequently dramatic improvement in the condition of the patient following an abreaction of this nature, it is hardly surprising that I found the subject so interesting and yet puzzling. What was going on, and what mechanism was at work?

Was abreaction only of use in the extremes of stress found only in battle trauma, or could it help in milder forms of anxiety? The answers to these questions came to me at a much later date when my knowledge of mental processes had greatly increased along with my experience in the use of hypnosis.

Of one thing I am certain, witnessing these events in my early years gave me, thereafter, the confidence to handle abreactions whenever they occurred. I was never afraid to encourage them nor to exploit them therapeutically as they arose under hypnosis.

Psychiatrists at that time used one of three methods to induce patients to abreact their wartime traumas. The first, 'ether abreaction', was done in a similar fashion to giving ether as an anaesthetic but using it in a much reduced concentration. Small quantities of liquid ether were dropped on to a Schimmelbusch face mask, and the fumes were inhaled by the patient. In the half-anaesthetized state that ensued the patient was asked to go back to the scene of the originating trauma and was encouraged to re-enact the events that had occurred (that is, 'abreact' these events). Ether, when inhaled, produces an excitatory mental state, and these patients often had to be restrained by force to prevent them causing damage to themselves or their attendants.

The second, 'pentothal abreaction', involved the slow intra-venous injection of a solution of sodium pentothal. As the patient became drowsy it was suggested to him that he re-live (abreact) his past traumatic history. Abreaction under pentothal was less excit-atory but it had less margin of error. Instead of abreacting, the patient often went through the drowsy stage too quickly and became unconscious.

These first two methods were certainly the treatment of choice at that time, but occasionally a visiting psychiatrist would use the third method, hypnosis. Under hypnosis the patient was asked to go back in time to the scene of stress and re-enact the events.

It seemed to me that the hypnotic method appeared physically less traumatic and, not unnaturally, it was favoured by the psychia-trist using it, who invariably considered the results obtained equal to those that were drug-induced.

In those days I was in no position to judge, but future experience has led me to believe that an excessive reaction to re-living past events is not a necessary criterion for a positive improvement to occur in the patient's condition. There is no doubt, however, that when a strong emotional re-living of past events occurs under hypnosis, improvement is almost certain to follow.

On the other hand, a patient may be seen to sob quietly as memories return. When the sobbing ceases and the patient is returned to the normal waking state, relief from anxiety may be equally profound and good progress follows.

If my attachment to Dr Strauss's out-patient clinic had streng-thened my interest in psychiatry, the following six months almost totally destroyed it. One of the results of the wartime dispersal of St Bartholomew's Hospital was that the final student medical and surgical units were located in part of an old Victorian mental hospital just outside St Albans. Hill-End Hospital, although beautifully situated in extensive, well-kept grounds, was itself a most depressing place in which to live. The walls of its long, inter-connecting corridors were covered with mournful, dark-brown or sickly green glazed tiles, and their concrete floors earily (and eerily) echoed the shuffling footsteps of their unfortunate inmates.

Admittedly, that section of the hospital taken over by Barts was a hive of industry and full of doctors, students, and scurrying young nurses in clean, fresh uniform going about their business with a lively chatter, but the contrast was too close to be ignored. That part of the hospital still occupied by the mental nursing staff and their patients was drab and mostly silent, only punctuated by the occasional cry of some tortured schizophrenic soul whose contact with the world had been reduced to an internal battle only known to himself. Every morning and afternoon a long line of the mental inmates in their dreary attire could be seen taking their constitutional shuffle around the grounds. The column walked slowly, usually in pairs, many with their heads bowed and all seemingly oblivious of their surroundings. In charge of them, and spaced at regular intervals, were the male nurses in their short white coats and long black trousers looking for all the world like human collie dogs maintaining the direction and momentum of their quasi-human flock. This long line of drugged automatons with severe mental afflictions was a really sad and depressing sight, and in those days very little in the way of treatment could be done for these patients.

I knew that, were I to take up psychiatry as a postgraduate subject, it would be necessary for me to gain experience in similar hospitals accommodating such patients. The thought of those years ahead was depressing and I became disillusioned.

I qualified MB BS in 1950 and the next two years were occupied with various house appointments at Bart's. One of these was as House Surgeon to the ENT department, the in-patient wards of which were still located at Hill-End. I thus inadvertently renewed my acquaintance with this hospital and, although I enjoyed the ward and theatre work, the mental section continued to depress me and I was pleased to return to out-patient work in Bart's at Smithfield.

Although the war ended in 1945 with the Japanese capitulation, conscription was still in force, and in 1952 I was called-up into the Royal Air Force. My final house job ended on the 30 June 1952, but my call-up date was not until mid-September of that year. This gave me ten weeks to fill in without any income. I could have continued in St Bartholomew's doing short (two-week) locums for various colleagues, but the pay was at the abysmal rate of £350 per annum, whereas in general practice a locum was paid three times as much! I not unnaturally decided to spend eight of the ten weeks as a locum tenens in general practice and then, with pockets full of unaccustomed wealth, spend the last two weeks on holiday in the South of France. This decision, made with no consideration other than the financing of a rather special holiday, turned out to be one of vital influence in shaping my future!

I became employed in two general practices. The first was for two weeks in a London commuter-belt, middle-class, semi-private practice where one of the partners in the practice was recuperating from a minor operation. This was lucky for me because he was only too willing to give me advice from his bed on the vicissitudes of life as a GP under the (then) new National Health Service. This, as it were 'supervised', introduction to general practice was of tremendous help to me when I took up my next locum tenens in what was a rapidly expanding practice on the edge of a new town being built on the outskirts of London. There were three partners in this practice, and each took two weeks' holiday one after the other, which effectively employed me for the remaining six weeks. The practice was so busy that I rarely saw the other doctors; I was left entirely to myself, loaned a car, and told to get on with it!

Coming after all those long years of hospital training and hospital employment, general practice was a complete revelation. I entered what appeared to me a totally new world of medicine where the patient was much more identifiable as an individual. That is not to say that hospitalized individuals were treated unsympathetically, or that their social history went unrecorded or unnoticed; it was more that Mrs A's verbal description of say, the house in which she lived, was insufficient to convey any emotional assessment of her character. It was not until one actually saw, entered, and smelt her house that a true reflection of any value was possible. Then again the mournful faces of her family and friends who had visited her when she was in hospital became more humanized: they also lived in houses, and rode bicycles, and went shopping, and drank in pubs, and queued for a cinema, and I came to know them as actual people.

The lump in the breast, the fractured head of femur, the acute appendicitis, were not the names in bold type on the diagnostic page of the hospital notes hanging at the end of the bed, they were much more.

Mrs Cartwright lived with her three children aged fourteen, twelve and ten, in a council house on a new estate. She found it very difficult to make ends meet on the war-widows pension. Her husband had been a merchant seaman. The ship in which he had sailed was part of an Atlantic convoy savaged by a U-boat pack in 1943. He was listed as 'missing presumed dead'. Her house was spotless and her children well behaved. She had been aware of the lump in her breast for some time but was terrified of it being a cancer and had delayed visiting the doctor. When she eventually plucked up the courage to do so it was too late: it was a cancer and it had spread to the glands in the axilla. When she realized her fate, the most important thing in her life was making sure that her children would be well cared-for after her death; the GP's job was to help her in this aim. The cancer (and its palliative treatment) became an almost minor issue.

The fractured neck of femur sustained by Granny when she slipped on her newly washed floor meant that her daughter had to leave her husband and family at home to fend for themselves while she camp-bedded in her mother's one-roomed flat. After three weeks an anonymous letter sent the daughter scurrying home. Granny's fracture had broken more than her bones and it took the combined efforts of two, previously unacquainted, GPs, 50 miles apart, to plaster up that marriage.

The acute appendicitis in the middle-aged bank clerk exposed his books to an unexpected scrutiny. The small amount of missing money which he had 'temporarily borrowed and was going to replace as soon as he was able' put his job in jeopardy. Written character references and the appearance of his GP in court explaining some family problems saved his job. In addition, the bank clerk's experience altered his whole demeanour for the better.

Perhaps the impression I gained in those few weeks that really set me thinking was the most noticeable relief from anxiety which showed on the faces of the family as they opened the door of their home to me in response to an urgent call. In almost all the cases I was a totally unknown stranger with an equal lack of knowledge of them. It was clear to me that it was the word 'doctor' that carried this enormous power of reassurance, and I was grateful to sense it. Being on my own without the customary back-drop of hospital support reduced my confidence at times to a sweaty low, but, to my great relief, the patients appeared not to notice this personal anxiety.

As confidence in myself gradually returned I realized that one of a GP's most valuable therapeutic assets is this in-built power of suggestion he carries with his stethoscope. I also realized that for every patient a GP ends up having to refer to a hospital, he will have successfully treated a hundred others. Furthermore, a large number of these patients would have responded to some form of medicine, the only possible action of which could have been that of a placebo.

It soon became obvious to me that, where stress, anxiety and so on produced symptoms of a psychosomatic nature, the GP's stock-in-trade in those days was the placebo, usually in the form of a 'nerve tonic'. As a result, practically everybody visiting the doctor expected to come away with a bottle of medicine suitably endorsed by verbal faith in its efficacy and strict written instructions for its consumption.

Provided the doctor's diagnosis was correct I saw no harm in this well-tried, highly effective, traditional method; at the same time I felt that ultra-strong suggestion in the form of hypnosis should give similar results without any possible side-effects from any chemicals in the placebo. I did not get a chance to test the theory in a general practice until I was demobbed from the Royal Air Force some two years later.

My conscription years were spent in Germany, the first half of which were in Berlin. I was the station medical officer at RAF Gatow and an ear, nose and throat graded specialist at the British Medical Hospital in Spandau.

Gatow was an important 'listening post' for monitoring Soviet Army movements in East Germany as well as being the airfield from which the tapes of the telephone-tapping section were flown back to the Zone. The individuals engaged in this work were classified as 'RAF Technicians' and were quartered within the station perimeter. They had been recruited because of their East European language abilities, and some had completed university short courses in Russian.

Their work involved spending long hours in front of powerful radio receivers in a constant state of concentration. Inevitably this led to a few cases of what could be termed 'mental exhaustion', the symptoms of which varied from an inability to sleep to the odd conversion symptom such as a hand tremor. I was able to relax these patients with the use of hypnosis, which was successful enough for them to complete their tour of duty.

Flight-Lieutenant James Penney, who was in charge of these technicians (Penney's men), was permanently short-staffed, and any who went sick just added to the burden of the others.

Both he and the commandant of Gatow, Wing-Commander F. Drury, rarely took time off, and it is a tribute to their industry and the care they took of their men that this very difficult monitoring section was one of the more successful sources of information available to Western intelligence at that time.

I left Berlin to open up the Ear, Nose and Throat Department of a new RAF hospital nearing completion at Rostrup in the Zone. This was a good experience for me and meant that I was virtually guaranteed an ENT registrar's post at a London teaching hospital when my National Service came to an end. But the Air Force had given me the time to consider the future. The National Health Service was in its infancy and a considerable state of flux; most consultant posts had been filled by those doctors whose careers had been interrupted by war service, and ENT was a very narrow field. I had very much enjoyed my brief encounter with general practice, and I particularly appreciated its wide medical scope, so when I was offered a salaried partnership in a practice where the senior partner was to retire within two years I decided to accept the offer.

It is not my intention to describe the life of a doctor in 1955 working in an expanding practice on the edge of a new town with totally inadequate hospital facilities. Suffice to say that the work was never-ending. It was not uncommon for each doctor to have thirty or more house calls in one day, not to mention the queues for morning and evening surgeries.

The families were all young and in the child-bearing period of their lives. Most babies were delivered at home. Many times I had to administer a general anaesthetic to a woman in labour and then perform the forceps delivery myself – there was no one else available! Almost all infectious diseases, including pneumonia, were treated at home – there were no hospital beds. The only exception was tuberculosis, and most counties had major hospitals confined solely to treating this disease.

Under these circumstances it was difficult to find the time to use hypnosis on one's patients; it was far easier to fall back on phenobarbitone and the ubiquitous placebo! Nevertheless I did manage to treat a few patients using hypnosis, despite some opposition from a quite unexpected quarter.

My senior partner was informed of a case I had treated with hypnosis which had turned out to be quite a spectacular success. Very briefly, the patient was a married male in his thirties who suffered with a disabling skin irritation diagnosed by the London Hospital as *Pityriarsis Lichenoides et Varioliformis* which they considered benign, harmless and usually self-limiting. He had suffered with this condition for over four years, had consulted various skin specialists and eventually ended up as an in-patient in the London Hospital with a fulminating staphylococcal infection of his skin. When he was discharged he remained under the London's Psychiatric Department as an out-patient for a year-and-a-half, during which time he did less than three months' work. The treatment he received from them was heavy sedation at night and tranquillizers during the day. He was quite incapable, under these conditions, of holding down a job. He lived with his wife and widowed mother-in-law in a council house. He hated the sight of his mother-in-law and resented being in a council house. Under hypnosis I rationalized his relationship with his mother-in-law and his surroundings, and suggested that all the energy he was using in resenting them would be better channelled into getting a job and earning enough money to buy a house of his own! This was primitive stuff in 1956 but it worked! After four sessions he was back at work without any skin irritation.

My senior partner called me into his drawing-room. He was extremely pleasant, almost apologetic, saying that he had no criticism of me personally or of my work but he was very worried about my using hypnosis. I quoted his own words back to him – that he had once told me that he considered general practice to be 80 per cent psychiatry. If that was indeed the case then hypnosis could be of great value to the practitioner. He replied that hypnosis smelt of the witch doctor, that I was playing around with forces *no one* knew anything about, that it was upsetting the local church (by that he meant the local Church of England vicar), and that as far as he was concerned he was unhappy about it. I knew him as a shrewd and competent general practitioner and respected his judgement in most matters. I dutifully toed the line until he retired a year later (1957), when I found myself as senior partner in my own practice.

Fifteen years later, on 8 May 1972, in the West Hall of the Royal Society of Medicine, I gave a lecture on the subject of hypnosis in general practice in which I quoted this incident with my senior partner. I ended the lecture with this statement:

> I still find an awful lot of prejudice against hypnosis particularly amongst the older consultants and general practitioners.
>
> But there is no doubt that, particularly in the last few years, as the very grave consequences of the massive drug and tranquillizer explosion become more obvious, that a greater part of the medical ear is being tuned into other methods of controlling the rising tensions and anxieties of the world we live in. I think in hypnotherapy we have a reasonably quick, normal, natural, safe method of helping patients overcome their own inadequacies without having to turn them into drug-addicts.

In the discussion that followed the lecture almost every doctor in the audience quoted similar intolerance they had personally experienced from colleagues in the profession.

It was at this precise point that I became determined to discover why this prejudice existed and how it could be eliminated. It soon became obvious to me that if there was *a satisfactory explanation of hypnosis in scientific terms*, it would go a long way to eliminating this prejudice. I felt that the most persuasive scientific terms would take the form of *a neurological explanation* of the phenomenon, and in researching this path I came across Roger Sperry's work on split-brained monkeys and humans. On 1 November 1982 I gave a lecture at the Royal Society of Medicine entitled 'Hypnosis and the right hemisphere', in which I put forward a possible explanation of the hypnotic phenomenon in neurological terms.

At the same time I outlined a practical method of analysing patients based on the supposition that a person in hypnosis is functioning mainly on their right hemisphere. I coined the term 'cameral analysis' for this method. This lecture was subsequently published; I quote from it in the chapters on theory later in this book.

Six years later, in my Presidential Address to the Section of Hypnosis and Psychosomatic Medicine on 3 October 1988 at the Royal Society of Medicine, I gave further evidence in support of my hypothesis and expanded on the method of cameral analysis. This lecture was subsequently published in the *Journal of the Royal Society of Medicine* (vol. 82, October 1989).

In the years from 1970 to the present day I have used hypnosis on hundreds of patients both in the National Health Service and in my private practice. During this same period I have given lecture demonstrations and held workshops in a medical capacity on many entirely professional courses held throughout the country.

My main aim throughout has been to adhere strictly to the scientific principle when evaluating the results of treatment involving the use of hypnosis compared with other treatments available for the same problem. I feel that only in this way can hypnosis become recognized and acceptable to the medical profession as a whole. I have tried to take out the magic and replace it with the mechanism. I have refuted, disproved and condemned the wild claims made by some so-called exponents of hypnosis who only serve to ridicule the subject in discerning eyes. The most important points I have persistently emphasized are first, that hypnosis is essentially an adjunct therapy to normal psychotherapy as taught in our medical schools and universities; secondly, individuals using hypnosis in the treatment of their patients must be well acquainted with normal and abnormal psychology as practised in general psychiatry, and should be capable of differentially diagnosing the psychoses from the neuroses as well as recognizing the organic origins of certain illnesses which may initially present as a mental disturbance. This offers little problem to medically qualified practitioners or those holding degrees or diplomas in psychology from recognized universities.

However, on the subject of lay psychotherapists there should be no compromise. Lay psychotherapists have inadequate or no training at all, they can be a danger to those of the public who become their patients, they are subject to no disciplinary body and they have no defence union to insure them.

Professor F. Frankel, of the Department of Psychiatry in the Harvard Medical School and a past President of the International Society of Hypnosis, is uncompromising when he voices the opinion of the latter organization concerning the membership and training of individuals in the use of hypnosis. He states: 'It is simply not possible to train in hypnosis someone who lacks an adequate clinical education, and expect that individual to become truly competent.'

As a result, the ISH restricts its entrants to physicians, clinical psychologists and others whose qualifications are without question. This society also considers it to be misguided and unethical for ISH members either to collaborate with or to train lay individuals using hypnosis.

I am reminded of Henry Rollin's discourse on charlatans in psychiatry.[2] His description of their danger to psychiatry could equally well apply to their use of hypnosis. He says words to the effect that they are those incompetent individuals who dabble with more fanaticism than understanding, more enthusiasm than common sense, and who exploit the ever-present demand for instant relief from mental anguish. So is the currency debased. When they jump on the bandwagon – they wreck it.

It is my firm belief that the use of hypnosis should become a naturally accepted form of medical treatment and more widely used in general practice. In the chapters that follow I hope to persuade members of the medical and para-medical profession to adopt hypnosis more universally and offer them a method (cameral analysis) incorporating its use in psychotherapy.

Part I

Theory

It is better to light a candle than curse the dark.

Chapter 1

A brief history of hemispheric lateralization

In 1980 a Nobel Prize was awarded to Professor Roger Sperry of the California Institute of Technology for his work on identifying specific functions of the brain which were lateralized either to the left or right cerebral hemispheres.[1] He concluded from this work that the human being consists of two people in the same body, he says:

> [We are] . . . two separate spheres of conscious awareness, that is two separate conscious entities running parallel in the same bony cranium each with its own sensations, perception, cognitive processes, learning experience, memories and so on.

This human division into left and right has been with us since humans first appeared on earth and was probably associated in the first place with handedness. Mythology abounds with examples of the universality of left versus right symbolism. From the most ancient of times, in virtually all cultures, laterality has had significant meaning attached to it, seemingly out of all proportion to its practical value. In the majority of male-dominant societies the right has been associated with good and the left with evil, with male and with female, with light and with darkness, with high and with low moral standing.

Where the societies have been matriarchal, however, the values have been reversed. Corballis, in a paper on laterality and myth (1980),[2] draws attention to the Isis cult of ancient Egypt where 'honour was given to Isis over Osiris, to mother over son, to night over day, and the Isis procession was headed by a priest carrying an image of the *left hand*'.

In neurological terms, mythology, by association with handedness, has identified the left hemisphere with dominance; philosophical, religious and judicial thought; and moral rectitude reflected in correct social behaviour within any given culture. This identification, as we shall see later, fits in well with the experimental findings of the Sperry team as they investigated their split-brained patients, as does mythology's condemnation of the right hemisphere as a Pandora's box of emotional, and illogical, devils.

Even Sperry's concept of two minds *in the same body* (bony cranium) was not new! 'Dualism'* – the concept of two minds – was well known to the Greeks and, of course, they had a word for it (ηετερως αυτως), which in translation means 'the other self'.

Later, when the Roman Empire absorbed the Greeks and everything Grecian, this 'other self' became the Roman 'alter ego'. For example, Ovid's famous dualistic *Deteriora sequor*, in which he actually looks at his other self with considerable disapproval, is similar indeed to the left hemisphere's moral criticism of certain right hemisphere behavioural demands. This 'other self', or 'alter ego', then, refers to both the clinical and cultural split in identity well recognized in human folklore, literature and poetry throughout the ages, from the *Odyssey* of Homer to the *Endymion* of Keats.

It was not until the eighteenth century, however, that dualism became almost a philosophical and literary obsession and was also recognized as a psychological phenomenon in the developing theories of mind prevalent at that time. This 'modern' concept of duality starts in the 1730s, when Anton Mesmer demonstrated the presence of 'another self' when he used 'animal magnetism' (now called 'hypnosis') to separate the alter ego. His demonstrations stimulated a behaviour pattern under hypnosis which was clearly different from the character of that individual in a normal 'waking' state. Suddenly, people could see another character in an altered state of consciousness but in the same body.

The theme exploded, particularly in the Romantic literature of the era, and German writer-philosophers such as Goethe, Kleist, Tieck, Hoffman and Jean Paul Richter were the first in the field to

---

* In the chapter 'A brief history of hemispheric lateralization', the words 'dualism' and 'duality' are used in their physical and psychological meaning in so far as they refer to the idea of two persons or personalities in a single body. This is in contradistinction to the philosophical meaning, which argues a physical and metaphysical (soul) component to existence. Sir John Eccles, however, approximates the two meanings to a certain extent in considering the left hemisphere to be the seat of religious comprehension (see Popper and Eccles, *The Self and its Brain*).[3]

explore this alter ego. It was Hoffman who, interestingly, identified the double with a somewhat dangerous part of the personality, and it was Richter who coined the term *doppelgänger* (Tymms 1949).[4]

In this the Romantic era of European history, the duality concept spread rapidly throughout the Western world, and perhaps the classic English versions in the literature of the time were Oscar Wilde's *The Picture of Dorian Gray* and Robert Louis Stevenson's *The Strange Case of Dr Jekyll and Mr Hyde*.

In both these novels a typical, logical, law-abiding, left hemisphere character is contrasted with an emotional, self-indulgent, sometimes murderous scoundrel, hell-bent on satisfying his lascivious desires, in fact a real right hemisphere renegade! There are many, many other literary examples on the same theme (Miller 1985).[5]

Charles Dickens was a great nineteenth-century dualist. In his last novel, *Edwin Drood* (the one he never finished), when drawing the character of Miss Twinkleton he states:

> As in some cases of drunkenness and in others of Animal Magnetism there are two states of consciousness which never clash, but each of which pursues its separate course as though it were continuous instead of broken (thus if I hide my watch when I am drunk, I must be drunk again before I can remember where), so Miss Twinkleton has two distinct and separate phases of being.

An interesting fact about Charles Dickens is that he was a very competent hypnotist. He was well acquainted with the concept of 'two selves in one body' from his interest in the hypnotic phenomenon. His great friend was none other than Dr John Elliotson.

Dr Elliotson was a scholar and President of the Royal College of Physicians in England, and arguably he was also one of the greatest exponents of the use of hypnosis in the early nineteenth century. In giving the Harveian Oration of 1846[6] Dr Elliotson extolled the value of hypnosis in producing anaesthesia, as well as its help in a variety of medical problems. Unfortunately this did not go down well with his colleagues and eventually led to the loss of his professorial chair at University College in London, a salutary lesson in the extent of hostility engendered by the subject amongst the medical fraternity of his era, a feeling which is sadly to this day all too prevalent.

Another nineteenth-century physician, perhaps the most intriguing of them all and yet barely acknowledged in his life-time, was Dr Arthur L. Wigan.[7] In 1844 he published a book entitled *The Duality of the Mind*, in which he set out to explain the duality concept in neurophysiological terms. He pre-empted Roger Sperry by over 100 years in so far as he postulated that the two cerebral hemispheres were capable of two separate and conflicting volitions. Furthermore, he went on to say that he considered the two hemispheres as two separate brains, one subordinate to the other, but nevertheless perfectly capable of acting independently of each other – Sperry's views almost word for word!

A French neurologist, Jean Baptiste Bouillard, in his treatise of 1825, asserted the possibility that we have a double intelligence, one on the right side of the brain and one on the left.

In 1840, the physician to Queen Victoria, Sir Henry Holland, put forward the idea that some mental illnesses might be due to 'incongruous action of the brain's two hemispheres'.[8]

In the last quarter of the nineteenth century Dr Frederick Myers, a Cambridge don and a founder-member of the British Society for Psychical Research, published an article on automatic writing[9] which was considered to be very important in the psychological field. In this article he raised the concept of the left hemisphere being more at the disposal of the 'waking' mind while the right hemisphere was more associated with the 'subconscious or subliminal self'. He came to this conclusion by drawing attention to the similarity of writing in patients who suffered from a right hemiplegia – that is, a paralysed right side of the body due to a malfunction of the left hemisphere from, for example, a stroke – and the automatic writing of subjects in an hypnotic or trance state. In both cases the words used were simple, often abbreviated, sometimes written in mirror-writing and often misspelt. *He concluded that trance states were right hemisphere-orientated.*

I believe this to be the first time that this theory was voiced, and it was taken very seriously by such world-renowned figures as William James, whose two volumes on *The Principles of Psychology*, first published in 1890,[10] became the first textbook on the then new subject of psychology. It was not until Roger Sperry's work on split-brained humans became known that the right hemisphere was again considered to be associated with the hypnotic state.

This time, 70 years later, it was neurological research that prompted its re-appraisal and that has enabled me to formulate a method of treatment of the neuroses based on hypnosis and the separate analysis of the two hemispheres.

Continuing with his theme, Myers followed his publication on automatic writing with a fascinating essay under the title of 'Multiplex personality' (Myers 1886).[11] In this essay he discusses a French physician's patient, a case of dual personality, Felida X, in whom two distinct characters emerged, neither of which was known to the other. One of these characters Myers considered to be Felida's 'normal self' and the other her 'somnambule or subliminal self', and he then went on to suggest that the subliminal self was regressive but artistically very creative – a description which fits well with that of the right hemisphere function. Interestingly, Myers follows this up by suggesting hypnosis as a treatment of choice in such cases, and suggests that hypnosis could re-arrange the 'looms of the mind' into a single, normally functioning pattern. In Chapter 9, p. 143, I describe a similar case of dual personality, who was the subject of a paper read to the Hypnosis Section of the Royal Society of Medicine in 1978.

Four years after Frederick Myers published his 'Multiplex personality' essay, a treatise in German written by Max Dessoir (1890)[12] was published under the title of *The Double Ego*, in which the subject of spontaneous somnambulism was discussed along with dipsychism and the hypnotic phenomenon. Dessoir was convinced that every single human individual was capable of being a double personality, each with the possibility of a separate existence yet both inextricably connected with a vast complex of association chains. His belief was engendered by his research and interest in hypnosis, and with its publication he became a nineteenth-century authority on the subject.

I cannot possibly end this brief history of dualism without mentioning Sigmund Freud. The idea of an 'unconscious mind' had been developing in eighteenth- and nineteenth-century thought ever since the phenomenon of animal magnetism had demonstrated the presence of an altered state of consciousness in human beings subjected to certain conditions. But as Lancelot Law Whyte points out in his book *The Unconscious before Freud*,[13] the concept of an unconscious mind has a distinguished ancestry which can be traced back to antiquity. Whyte states:

As Margetts[14] has said, 'Almost since the dawn of civilization man has had an inkling of understanding that mind activity outside of our waking consciousness does exist.' This could be proved by citations from the Indian Upanishads, from ancient Egypt and Greece, and, I believe, from many other civilizations.

All the greatest human documents, such as the Old and New Testaments and the writings of Plato, Dante, Cervantes, and Shakespeare, reveal this understanding.

As the method of investigating mental phenomena advanced from phrenology to the new subject of psychology, so the idea of the *alter idem* of an unconscious mind became a real possibility to many of the researchers in this field, and Freud, of course, was one of them. Nevertheless, it was Pierre Janet (1859–1947)[15] who was the first nineteeth-century physician to write about the concept of an unconscious mind, although he coined the term 'subconscious' to describe it. Janet's concept was later to be taken up by Freud and renamed 'the unconscious'. Both Jung and Adler were later to acknowledge their debt to Janetian thinking as their own theories developed (Ellenberger 1970).[16] I have already mentioned Frederick Myers, who had suggested that there was a *subliminal personality* which was both creative but at the same time regressive. William James in his book *The Principles of Psychology*[17] wrote of a 'hidden self'.

It was in Dr A. Liébault's clinic in Nancy that Freud himself became convinced of the presence of an unconscious mind.

He witnessed a post-hypnotic suggestion carried out by a patient who, on later questioning by Freud, had no knowledge of why she had performed this act but nevertheless made up a plausible explanation totally different from the real reason. Freud concluded that, to the patient, the real reason must be unconscious and/or repressed.

The whole foundation of psychoanalysis lay in these two concepts, the presence of an unconscious mind and the theory of repression. Freud's debt to hypnosis was largely ignored by him in his life-time. (Freud's theory, of course, was pure dualism, as indeed was that of Jung with its extrovert and introvert, its shadow self and its bad double.)

In America as well, at the end of the nineteenth century, dualism and hypnosis were bedfellows, and the use of hypnosis as a form of treatment was very popular. Such East Coast professors as Wier Mitchell and Morton Prince as well as William James wrote copiously on the subject, and used the phenomenon of hypnosis as evidence for dualism as had their European counterparts; some of their more fascinating patients exhibiting this dualistic somnambulism (for example, the Rev. Ansel Bourne and Mary Reynolds) are now part of the annals of American medical history.

After this very brief historical review we come to the twentieth century, and specifically to the last twenty years. What evidence have we now that was not available in the nineteenth century that warrants the resurrection of the duality theory? What has come about that has led to an empirical theory, first suggested by Dr Arthur Wigan in 1844, being re-stated almost word for word 150 years later by a research neurologist, Professor Roger Sperry, working at the California Institute of Technology?

Furthermore, what is it that has made the recent theory appear to be totally new and original and of such importance that a Nobel Prize and world-wide acclaim has been its reception?

I will try to answer these questions in the light of research into hemispheric specificity and relate the findings to the hypnotic phenomenon.

Chapter 2

The relationship between hypnosis and the right hemisphere

I have tried to show in my chapter on the history of hemispheric lateralization that, certainly from the nineteenth century and probably before, there has existed a body of individuals practising mainly in the fields of neurology, psychiatry and psychology, who have considered the hypnotic phenomenon to be a right hemisphere-orientated task. I am certainly one of them, and my experience in the use of hypnosis in the treatment of the psychoneuroses has led me to formulate a method based on this hypothesis which, for me at least, has produced good results over the years.

That the state of 'hypnosis' is associated with mental functioning in the right hemisphere is still *an hypothesis* and will remain one despite some convincing evidence in its favour. Nevertheless, as time goes on and more sophisticated research into brain-function takes place, from the evidence we have at the moment I feel it can only be supportive.

In this chapter I will take a critical look at the right hemisphere and its relationship to hypnosis. It will be shown how this hypothesis has been developed and why the whole concept of the right hemisphere is so important in the practical – that is, the clinical – use of hypnosis.

For the sake of clarity and simplicity, only right-handed adults are considered at this moment; they constitute 95 per cent of the populace and have their speech centre largely confined to their left cerebral hemisphere. I should also point out that the nerve fibres conducting messages to and from the brain cross over before entering and after leaving the skull. This means that the right side of the brain controls the left side of the body and, similarly, the left brain controls the right side. There are also pathways that do not cross (ipsilateral), but their function is marginal.

In October 1981, the Nobel Prize for Medicine and Physiology was jointly awarded to three researchers; two of them, Professor David Hubel and Professor Torsten Wiesel of Harvard Medical School, for their work on visual perception. The important part of their work shows that the visual cortex's ability to interpret impulses from the retina is developed after birth, and that it is vitally important for a rich variety of visual stimuli to be present during that period of the baby's development, otherwise permanent impairment of visual function can result. Interestingly, this could be interpreted as support for Gerald Edelman's 'theory of neuronal group selection', but for the moment Hubel and Wiesel's discovery is purely of academic interest and I mention it only in the context of the third recipient, who was Professor Roger Sperry. It was the latter's work in discovering the functional specialization of the two cerebral hemispheres that earned him the Nobel Prize and stimulated my interest in its application to hypnosis. Before considering Professor Sperry's work in more detail I think it is useful to look at what is known about how the human brain works and how it has evolved.

P.D. MacLean (1955)[1] and his co-workers in the 1970s (MacLean 1970)[2,3] came to the conclusion that the human brain is, in fact, the evolutionary result of three overlapping, basic brain types. Our brain today consists of these three different types joined together in one structure, which they called the 'Triune brain', and the highly intriguing and interesting factors are that each one has its own motor system, its own subjectivity, its own sense of time and space, its own special intelligence; and they all three differ entirely in their own neurochemical and microscopic structure. In addition, although the three types of brain are inter-connected and functionally inter-dependent, there is evidence, within certain limits, that they can operate independently of one another (MacLean 1976).[4]

These three brains are:

1 the reptilian brain (Figure 2.1);
2 the paleomammalian brain, also known as the limbic brain, or the visceral brain (Figure 2.2);
3 the neomammalian brain, also known as the neocortex (Figure 2.3).

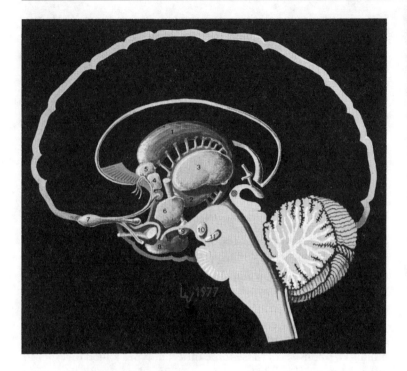

A diagrammatic representation of the structures involved in the function of this, the most ancient cerebrotype, responsible for elementary functions vital for survival.

1 Caudate nucleus	7 Olfactory bulb
2 Putamen and globus pallidus	8 Amygdala
3 Thalamus	9 Mammillary bodies
4 Septal nuclei	10 Red nucleus
5 Nucleus acumbens	11 Substantia nigra
6 Hypothalamus	12 Indusium griseum

Figure 2.1 The reptilian brain

Source: L. Valzelli (1980) *An Approach to Neuroanatomical and Neurochen Psychophysiology*, p. 7. By kind permission of Butterworth-Heinemann, Oxford.

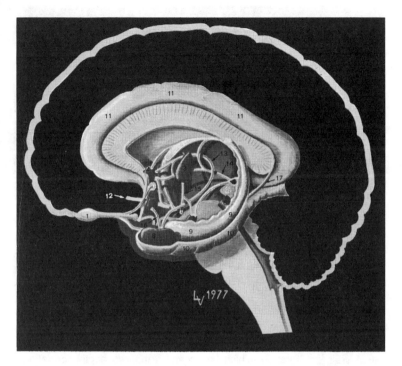

A diagrammatic representation of the structures involved in the function of this, the early mammalian brain, consisting of the limbic system surrounding the brain-stem and enclosing the reptilian brain. It adds the affective-emotive dimension to behaviour.

1 Olfactory bulb
2 Septal nucleus
3 Anterior section of the thalamus
4 Nucleus of the habenula
5 Mammillary bodies
6 Periaqueductal grey substance
7 Interpeduncular nucleus
8 Amygdala
9 Hippocampus

10 Hippocampal gyrus
11 Cingulate gyrus
12 Medial forebrain bundle
13 Stria terminalis
14 Stria medullaris
15 Mammillothalamic tract
   (Bundle of Vicq d'Azyr)
16 Broca's diagonal band
17 Fasciola cinerea

Figure 2.2 The paleomammalian brain or the limbic brain

Source: L. Valzelli (1980) *An Approach to Neuroanatomical and Neurochemical Psychophysiology*, p. 11. By kind permission of Butterworth-Heinemann, Oxford.

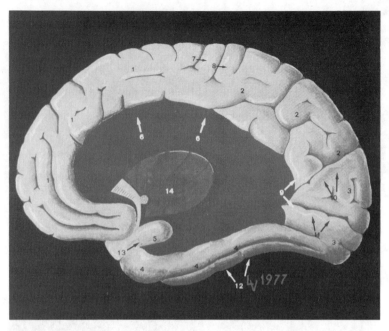

A diagrammatic representation of the structures involved in the function of this, the neomammalian brain or neocortex. It is phylogenetically the latest brain proliferation, which has covered the two earlier formations and reaches its greatest development in man and is exemplified by the presence of language areas.

1 Frontal lobe	8 Central sulcus (fissure of Rolando)
2 Parietal lobe	9 Subparietal sulcus
3 Occipital lobe	10 Parieto-occipital sulcus
4 Temporal lobe	11 Calcarine sulcus
5 Uncus	12 Collateral sulcus
6 Cingulate gyrus	13 Rhinal sulcus
7 Precentral sulcus	14 Insula of Reil

Figure 2.3 The neomammalian brain or the neocortex

Source: L. Valzelli (1980) *An Approach to Neuroanatomical and Neurochem. Psychophysiology*, p. 13. By kind permission of Butterworth-Heinemann, Oxford.

THE REPTILIAN BRAIN (Figure 2.1)

This is the most ancient brain and is responsible for elementary functions vital for survival, such as choice of, and defence of, territory within which the subject carries out his life-sustaining activities; for example, hunting, competition, social rank and mating (MacLean 1972).[5]

Its behaviour is strikingly rigid and ritualized and very stereotyped, showing compulsive patterns which have been genetically transmitted to govern imitative behaviour, such as the imprinting phenomenon at birth (Lorenz 1937)[6] and forms of behaviour where rough imitations of shapes of birds, colours, and so on stimulate defence or acceptance behaviour (Tinbergen 1951).[7]

THE PALEOMAMMALIAN OR LIMBIC OR VISCERAL BRAIN (Figure 2.2)

This early mammalian brain consists of that system (the limbic system) surrounding the brain-stem and enclosing the reptilian brain.

Its function is that it adds the affective-emotive dimension to behaviour, thus modulating information from the environment and colouring it with emotion, giving us a much wider range of more flexible behaviour for self and species preservation (Fulton 1951),[8] (MacLean 1958),[9] (Papez 1937).[10] In addition, it not only receives information from the external environment via its visual, auditory, olfactory, gustatory and skin sensors, but also adds somatic or visceral senses.

THE NEOMAMMALIAN BRAIN OR THE NEOCORTEX (Figure 2.3)

This is the rapidly proliferating brain which has covered the two earlier formations and reaches its greatest development in man.

It differs from the other two in two vitally important factors. First, Valzelli (1980)[11] states:

> It has no direct information channels of its own from the environment. As a result all outside environmental information and all inner or visceral information arrives at the neocortex for processing via the two other brains and it has already been modulated by them, in particular, of course, by the emotional

colouring of the limbic system. In man, therefore, the neo-cortex is the site of abstract thoughts, reflection, reasoning both mathematical and philosophical, cognition, understand-ing, invention, analysis and synthesis, creative imagination, and intuition.

Secondly, in humans and humans alone, it has developed lan-guage areas in the neocortex. These areas in adult humans are confined mainly to one hemisphere, and in 95 per cent of cases this is the left hemisphere. The right hemisphere is devoid of any major speech areas and as such is only capable of communicating in this medium with an extremely limited vocabulary. The vitally import-ant point about the fact that the speech areas in adult humans are virtually unilateral is that it has historically stimulated the concept of *lateralization*.

As work progressed in this field and increasing numbers of lateralized processes were demonstrated, these were all considered to be the result of verbal lateralization, but it has now become increasingly clear that both hemispheres exhibit specializations, and Professor Marcel Kinsbourne (1978)[12] suggests that the ques-tion 'Are there any cognitive functions that are asymmetrically represented?' should be changed. We should now ask, 'Are there any cognitive functions that *are not* asymmetrically represented?'

Let us now look more closely at Professor Sperry's work.

In the 1950s, Roger Sperry and his assistant, Ronald Myers, working at the California Institute of Technology, began a series of split-brain experiments on living animals. They started with cats, and cut all connections between the left and right halves of the brains of these creatures. Later they repeated these experi-ments on monkeys. Their first extraordinary finding was that these animals, after they had recovered from the operation, appeared to behave to all intents and purposes in a normal fashion. Nevertheless, to their astonishment, they were able to train the monkeys as if they had two, totally separate, brains. An apparatus was designed so that the left and right hemispheres of the brain of these animals could be individually stimulated by a figure pro-jected on a screen placed in front of them. In this way they were able to train the animal to execute the same task in response to two differing stimuli. The right paw (activated by the left motorcortex) could be trained to push a lever down to obtain food when the animal saw an 'X' in front of it. The left paw (right cortex) could be trained to push the same lever down only when it saw an 'O' and would totally ignore the 'X' (Sperry 1956).[13] The human breakthrough to these experiments came in late 1962 when Vogel and Bogen operated upon a patient in Los Angeles in an attempt to stop his almost continuous epileptic seizures (Bogen 1962).[14] They cut his corpus callosum and thus isolated his two hemispheres, making him into a split-brain man (see Figure 2.4 and 2.5). This operation was extremely successful and has been performed on many other patients since. Of course, Sperry could not wait to get his hands on these patients, and he and Michael Gazzaniga devised ingenious experiments which allowed isolated communication with one hemisphere or the other.

In one such experiment (Figure 2.6) the split-brain patient sits in front of a screen underneath which is a table with various easily recognizable, small household articles. These articles cannot be seen by the patient but he is able to examine them with his hands. A picture of a spoon is projected on to the *left side* of the screen, which means that only his right hemisphere sees the image. When asked what he saw, he verbally states that he saw nothing on the screen. Nevertheless, his left hand (controlled by his right hemisphere) is able to pick out a spoon from a group of objects while he is still verbally insisting that he saw nothing. On the other hand, if the name of the object is flashed on the *right side* of the screen the patient can both pick it out and also describe it in words.

If dissimilar objects are projected at the same time on both the left- and right-hand side of the screen, the patient will pick out what he saw on the left with his left hand (say, a pencil) and what he saw on the right with his right hand (say, a ball) *without being aware of any conflict*. If you ask this patient why his left hand picked out an object which differs from both the choice of his right hand and his verbal affirmation of that choice, he blandly dismisses the question by a remark such as 'Well I must have done it unconsciously,' or 'I have simply no idea' (Sperry 1968).[15]

Another experiment done by M.S. Gazzaniga and J.E. Le Doux (1978)[16] (Figure 2.7) shows simultaneous presentation of two different tasks, one to each hemisphere, of patient P.S.

In describing this split-brain experiment Gazzaniga states:

Where the snow scene was presented to the RIGHT Hemisphere and a chicken claw to the LEFT, P.S. quickly and dutifully responded correctly by choosing a picture of a chicken

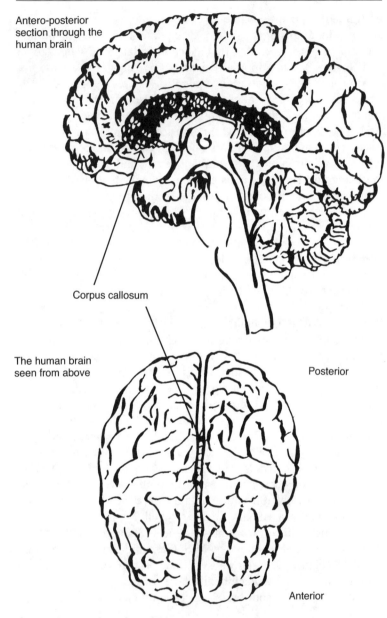

Antero-posterior
section through the
human brain

Corpus callosum

The human brain
seen from above

Posterior

Anterior

Figure 2.4 The corpus callosum: the interhemispheric conducting fibres
severed in the split-brain operation

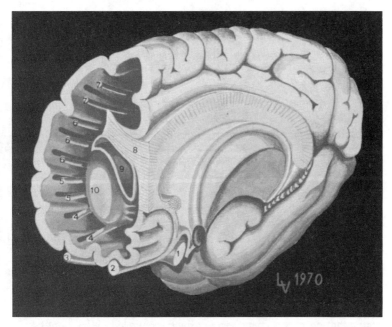

It is from the activation of the Reticular Formation by the Superior Frontal Gyrus via its Front-Reticular Projection Pathways that inhibition of global awareness is induced. Professor Wyke's theory postulates that hypnosis is the result of reducing the state of global awareness to one sensory input source, namely that of the voice of the hypnotist.

1 Optic chiasm
2 Olfactory bulb
3 Optic nerve
4 Cingulate afferences
5 Sensory afferences

6 Premotor afferences
7 Motor afferences
8 Corpus callosum
9 Lateral ventricle
10 Head of Caudate nucleus

Figure 2.5 A three-dimensional representation of the corpus callosum, severed in the split-brain operation, and showing its anatomical relationship to the frontal lobe (right)

Source: L. Valzelli (1980) *An Approach to Neuroanatomical and Neurochemical Psychophysiology*, p. 37. By kind permission of Butterworth-Heinemann, Oxford.

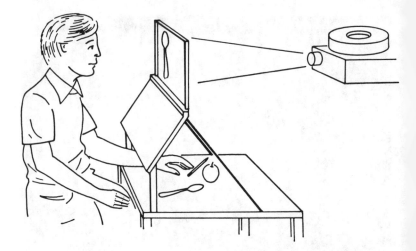

The split-brain patient sits in front of a screen underneath which is a table with various small household articles. These articles cannot be seen by the patient but he is able to examine them with his hands. A picture of a spoon is projected on to the *left side* of the screen, which means only his right hemisphere sees the image. When asked what he saw, he verbally states that he saw nothing. His left hand, controlled by his right hemisphere, is able to pick out a spoon from a group of objects while he is still verbally insisting he that he saw nothing.

Figure 2.6 Functions of the two hemispheres

Source: Adapted from T.R. Blakeslee (1980) *The Right Brain.* Macmillan, London, with permission.

from a series of four cards with his right hand and a picture of a shovel from a series of four cards with his left hand. The subject was then asked 'What did you see?'

He replied, 'I saw a chicken claw and picked the chicken and you have to clean out the chicken shed with a shovel.'

In trial after trial we saw this kind of response. The left hemisphere could easily and accurately identify why it had picked the answer, and then subsequently, and without batting an eyelid, it would incorporate the right hemisphere's response into the framework. Whilst we knew exactly why the right hemisphere had made its choice, the left hemisphere could merely guess. Yet the left hemisphere did not offer its suggestion in a guessing vein, but rather a statement of fact as to why that card had been picked.

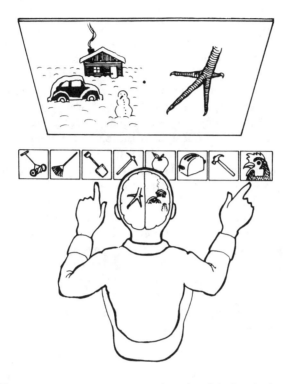

Where the snow scene was presented to the right hemisphere and a chicken claw to the left, P.S. quickly and dutifully responded correctly by choosing a picture of a chicken from a series of four cards with his right hand. The subject was then asked, 'What did you see?' He replied, 'I saw a chicken claw and picked the chicken and you have to clean out the chicken-shed with a shovel.'

In trial after trial Gazzaniga and Le Doux saw this kind of response. The left hemisphere could easily and accurately identify why it had picked the answer, and then subsequently, and without batting an eyelid, it would incorporate the right hemisphere's response into the framework. Although they knew exactly why the right hemisphere had made its choice, the left hemisphere could merely guess. Yet the left hemisphere did not offer its suggestion in a guessing vein, but rather a statement of fact as to why that card had been picked.

Figure 2.7 Tasks of each hemisphere

Source: M.S. Gazzaniga and J.E. Le Doux (1978) *The Integrated Mind*, p. 149, Figure 42. Plenum Press, New York.

This fascinating observation by Gazzaniga has a very important bearing on the (previously mentioned) hypnotic phenomena observed by Freud in Liébault's clinic in Nancy, and which led Freud directly to formulate his theory of repression.

In the clinic, a patient was given the post-hypnotic suggestion (while under hypnosis) that when she came out of the hypnotic trance she was to open an umbrella which was lying on the table beside her. She did this exactly as had been suggested to her under hypnosis. Freud then questioned the patient as to why she had found it necessary to carry out this act. The patient had apparently no idea whatsoever, but made up a story to fit her action. She made up this story to explain why she had to put up the umbrella, precisely as a split-brained person does when trying to explain why his left hand picked up one object, but verbally stated it was another.

From this Freud deduced that certain facts were being unconsciously repressed by this patient. In the light of Gazzaniga's patient, however, it would also support the contention that, when we hypnotize a patient, what we are doing is limiting their mode of consciousness to the right hemisphere by inhibition of the left. We know this is neurologically possible by stimulation of the inhibiting potentials of the caudal end of the reticular formation of the brain-stem (Wyke 1960).[17]

To enlarge on this a little further; Dr Barry Wyke's theory is that hypnosis is 'An altered state of consciousness in which the global awareness of the individual is reduced to one sensory input source, namely that of the voice of the hypnotist.' He then goes on to postulate that 'This is neurologically possible by activation of the inhibitory fibres of the caudal end of the brain-stem reticular formation and that this activation stimulus comes from the superior frontal gyrus via its fronto-reticular projection pathways.'

It is important at this point to quote again Professor Sperry's (1968)[18] observations on the split-brain individual. Professor Sperry stated:

> In the split-brain syndrome we deal with two separate spheres of conscious awareness, that is two separate conscious entities running parallel in the same bony cranium, each with its own sensations, perceptions, cognitive processes, learning experiences, memories and so on.

A variety of research workers, including Howard Gardner (1977)[19] of Boston, have made extensive studies in patients suffering from damaged brains, such as from strokes, tumours, or injuries, all of which have been complementary to Sperry's work on split-brain patients. Their work and that of Professor Sperry has all shown that specific qualities become lateralized to one hemisphere or the other. For instance, there is an experiment on a split-brain patient in which the patient looks at a scrambled drawing of a geometric shape and tries to match it to one of three solid shapes, placed out of sight, but which he can feel with either one hand or the other. *It was found that only the left hand (that is the right brain) could solve this problem.*

This and other experiments show that the right hemisphere copes with predominantly spatial problems, whereas the left side has a very good linear logic and, of course, language ability. This spatial property of the right hemisphere is vital in sport and in recognizing faces, and so on. Whereas the left brain can verbally 'see' how to play tennis, it cannot spatially computerize the trajectory of the ball in the actual game of tennis. A good tennis player is playing almost entirely through his right hemisphere. How often has the expression been heard, 'He is playing as if in a dream' (as in the hypnotic state)?

In 1974,[20] Tim Gallwey, a professional tennis coach, wrote an immediate best-seller called *The Inner Game of Tennis*. Gallwey's theory was that each person's mind contains a verbal self-one and a non-verbal, unconscious self-two, which actually plays the game. When teaching students, Gallwey avoids all verbal communications wherever possible and relies entirely on visual images, thus teaching the correct hemisphere in the language it understands. The success of this non-verbal technique fits in well with the observations by Professor Sperry of the separate functions of the two hemispheres, and as such is predictable.

A very enterprising artist, Betty Edwards (1979),[21] teaching in California State University, came across Professor Sperry's work and predicted that, by concentrating on teaching techniques designed to force her students to use the right hemisphere, she should be able to improve their artistic ability.

Her results were outstanding and her 'cognitive shift' method of teaching has made a profound impact on art schools throughout the world. Her book, *Drawing on the Right Side of the Brain*, is also a best-seller.

At this point we have *the first whisper of 'cameral analysis'*.

If we assume that the altered state of consciousness seen under hypnosis is in fact a right hemisphere-orientation, then any technique which uses the skills or 'language' of the right hemisphere for communication should produce a greater understanding of the right hemisphere's (largely emotional) problems.

By encouraging patients, both in and out of hypnosis, to express their anxieties in, say, artistic form – for instance, drawing, painting and so on – their problems should become more obvious to the therapist. Furthermore, this non-verbal act of expression by the patient has, in itself, a therapeutic value. Other techniques using song, dance, poetry, music and so forth should show similarly good results. It is interesting to note that Mesmer himself played music to his patients while giving therapeutic suggestions under hypnosis (Critchley and Henson 1977).[22]

All of these techniques have been used, either in isolation or some combination, by one therapist or another over the years. By combining them with the separate analysis of each hemisphere, both insight into patients' problems and a therapy for resolving them are joined together in one therapeutic method under the heading of cameral analysis.

To revert to the split-brained patient, it has been shown that the spatial ability of the right hemisphere enables recognition of faces. It has been found that people with complete loss of the right hemisphere cannot recognize individuals unless they are actually named.

Another factor in these patients with complete loss of the right hemisphere is that, although they know who they are, their visual recognition of their whereabouts is impaired. The third factor is that they have a total loss of any emotional recognition.

The left brain is totally unable to recognize any anger or enthusiasm in faces or voice intonation. This leads to the concept that the brain can have two different interpretations of the same incident (Galin 1974),[23] a concept of great importance, which is discussed at length later in the chapter. A BBC television programme on the subject of hypnosis given by Professor Frankel quite accidentally illustrated this phenomenon, of the possibility of *two interpretations of the same event*, very admirably.

Professor F. Frankel of Harvard Medical School hypnotized a female volunteer. He asked her, under hypnosis, to go back in time to a happy event in her childhood. She went back to this event and then started crying! The event that had verbally been presented to her for months and months as a happy event was the birth of her sister. When this event actually occurred it turned out to be a nightmare for the patient at that age. Her mother suddenly developed a severe pain, called the ambulance and was whisked off to hospital, leaving the patient all alone and terrified until the evening when her father returned! This incident in her mind had two interpretations; the verbal left hemisphere's acceptance of a happy event and the emotional right hemisphere's actual terror on that day.

This woman was not a split-brain patient but a normal person under hypnosis – that is, as I believe, working primarily in a right hemisphere mode.

The hypnotist's verbal request put her on target, as it were, for a *verbal* happy event which in this case did not coincide with an *emotional* happy event. Had she not been in hypnosis she would have no doubt related the birth of her sister to the audience with apparently genuine pleasure!

Phobic patients exhibit the same phenomenon. How often have we heard phobic patients verbally stating with emphasis that there is no rhyme or reason for them to be afraid of going, say, into a large store. Yet when they do, they panic and have to run out.

In these patients' minds there are two interpretations of the large store: (a) the verbal left hemisphere's logical one, which sees it as a harmless store, and (b) the emotional right hemisphere's one, which perhaps remembers the horror of being lost, as a child, in such a store. These patients as they enter the store fail to retain their left hemisphere logical mode, flip over onto a right hemisphere emotional mode, promptly panic and rush out.

By revealing and releasing emotional memory of the right hemisphere under hypnosis and bringing it to terms with the logical left such phobias should theoretically be controlled.

Perhaps one of the most significant and far-reaching factors to come out of the research on split-brain individuals is that, although the two hemispheres behave like two separate individuals, only one of the two will give the answer to any given problem. The experiment which illustrated this phenomenon was performed by Jerre Levy and Colwyn Trevarthen (1977)[24] when split-brain patients were given tests of elementary linguistic ability (see Figures 2.8a, 2.8b and 2.8c).

Using a modified two-channel tachistoscope, chimeric figures in the form of composite words were projected onto a screen in front of the patient. (A tachistoscope is a binocular gadget designed to confine views seen to the right of the midline to the visual cortex of the left hemisphere, and vice versa.) This meant that the patient's

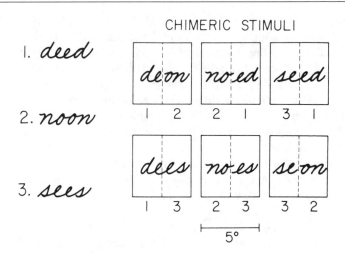

Figure 2.8a Chimeras and choices for palindrome test

Source: J. Levy and C. Trevarthen (1977) *Brain*, 100. By permission of Oxford University Press.

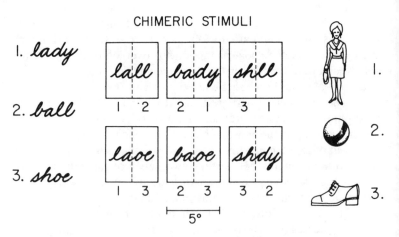

Figure 2.8b Chimeras and choices for word–picture matching

Source: J. Levy and C. Trevarthen (1977) *Brain*, 100. By permission of Oxford University Press.

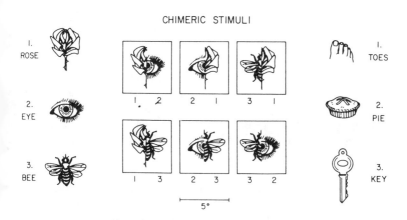

Figure 2.8c Chimeras and choices for rhyming test

Source: J. Levy and C. Trevarthen (1977) *Brain*, 100. By permission of Oxford University Press.

right hemisphere saw only that part of the word appearing on the left half of the screen and the left hemisphere that part appearing on the right of the screen. The chimeric figure 'DEON' made out of the palindromes (that is, words spelling the same left to right and right to left), 'DEED' and 'NOON', when projected on the screen would be seen by the right hemisphere as 'DE' and the left as 'ON'. Thus, if the patient were to be asked to match what was seen on the screen with the two normal words, his left brain would choose 'NOON' and his right brain 'DEED'. The eventual choice would therefore indicate to the experimenter exactly which hemisphere was answering.

The first task was matching words by *visual identity* (Figure 2.8a). Six chimeric figures were made from three short palindromes. As each was projected, the patient was asked to *point* to one of the three words 'DEED', 'NOON' and 'SEES' placed on the table in front of him. *He was not allowed to speak, only to point.*

First the left hand was used and then the right. The results showed that over 90 per cent of the answers were made by the right hemisphere, which indicated that it was using its pattern recognition ability by simply matching the fragmented word to a similar pattern.

When the patients were asked to *say* what word was seen, the results were reversed and the left hemisphere dominated.

The second task was *word/picture* matching: semantic decoding (Figure 2.8b). In this test, chimeras made of 'LADY', 'BALL' and 'SHOE' were presented, but the patient was required, without speaking or moving his mouth, to point to a picture corresponding with the word chosen from a group of three pictures, each depicting one of the words. The results showed a significant bias in favour of performing the task with the left hemisphere. This is explained by the lack of pattern similarity, which had the effect of confusing the right hemisphere, whereas the left hemisphere read the half-words as completed words and could then relate them to the pictures.

When giving their answers in the above two experiments, the patients seemed totally unconcerned with the information from the hemisphere they had ignored. The hemisphere not answering appeared simply to shut down in favour of the one with the greater potential to solve the problem. This would suggest that in normal, everyday life, the dominant hemisphere should be the one best suited to give the reply. In the majority of decisions I am sure this ideal situation pertains, but where the problem is complicated with emotion, a correct logical result could be the one inhibited. As Dr Ewin points out in his Foreword, 'when the will and imagination are at odds, the imagination tends to win'.

Another significant factor brought out by this Levy/Trevarthen experiment was the identifying of a specific capability apparently confined to one hemisphere. Results from the third task suggested the presence of a phonetic encoder possessed only by the left hemisphere.

This third task was to test the ability of the hemispheres to *rhyme (phonetic similarity)* (Figure 2.8c). The patient was instructed not to speak, but to indicate silently, by pointing, which of the three objects had a name that rhymed with the name of the object seen through the tachistoscope. The objects were pictures of toes, a pie, and a key and the projected chimeras were composite pictures of a rose, an eye and a bee. The result of this test showed that the left hemisphere was vastly superior to the right, which displayed little, if any, ability to rhyme. The researchers concluded that the right hemisphere lacks a phonetic analyser that can also generate phonetic images.

From these three tests it becomes obvious that the left hemisphere has vastly superior linguistic skills but the right hemisphere has dominance over the left where *solely* visual matching is concerned. This finding supports the ability of the right hemisphere over the left in the recognition of facial features, which brings me to the difference in personalities between the theoretical left and right hemisphere persons.

There are two methods that can be used to isolate one hemisphere from the other in normal individuals. The first is the Wada test. Sodium amytal is injected into the left or right carotid artery (Wada 1949)[25], and temporary anaesthesia is produced in the hemisphere of the selected side. The test was developed to determine which side of the brain controlled speech in patients about to undergo brain surgery.

The second method is by applying electroconvulsive therapy (ECT) to one hemisphere only, knocking it out temporarily, thus temporarily giving the other hemisphere the whole stage, as it were.

Vadim L. Deglin (1976)[26] a leading Russian neurophysiologist working at the I.M. Sechenov Institute of the USSR Academy of Sciences in St Petersburg, has carried out studies on patients receiving unilateral ECT. From the large numbers of patients studied he has been able to draw up a composite picture of the personality and ability of each hemisphere.

Taking the left hemisphere person first: after unilateral ECT to the right hemisphere, this hemisphere becomes temporarily inoperative and leaves mental activity only in the left. The left hemisphere becomes more active as a result of being freed from inhibitory competition of the right, and this is most noticeable in the patient's speech.

Thomas Blakeslee (1980)[27] has very adequately summarized Vadim's finding as follows:

The left hemisphere person

The patient becomes more talkative sometimes to an excessive degree. His vocabulary becomes richer and more varied and his answers are more extensive and detailed. At the same time his intonation is less expressive; it is monotonous, colourless and dull. His voice itself acquires a kind of nasal twang, or becomes unnatural, as though the patient were barking. A similar defect is observed in the patient's sensitivity to tone of voice. The left hemisphere by itself is unable to detect such things as anger, playfulness or enthusiasm as communicated by intonation of the voice. Even the difference between male and female voice is often undetectable without the help of the right brain.

When tape recordings of natural sounds such as coughing, laughter, snoring and breaking surf are played, the patient either cannot identify them or takes a long time to identify them.

Often the left hemisphere will attempt to classify the sound rather than identify it. For example, instead of saying, 'that's a dog barking' he will say 'that's an animal'.

Often the classification is wrong, but the effort to classify is symptomatic of the left hemisphere approach. Another defect that occurs is the inability to sing or to recognise well-known tunes. When asked to hum along with the music, the patient will generally hum the wrong notes and eventually end up just tapping out the rhythm without the melody.

Visual perception is also impaired without the help of the right hemisphere.

The patient will typically fail to notice missing details on uncomplicated pictures. For example, a pig with no tail, or spectacles with no earpieces will go unnoticed. When asked to match pairs of simple geometric figures such as triangles, squares, etc., the patient is unable to do it if the figures are covered with confusing coloured or striped sectors. This is the classic problem of not being able to 'see the forest for the trees'. Though the patient can name the hospital, ward number, and other such verbal details, his visual recognition of his where-abouts is clearly impaired. He looks in bewilderment at the consulting room to which he has been a frequent visitor and says he has never been there before.

While he can easily memorise and recite new verbal material, he is unable to memorise and identify shapes that are not easily given a verbal label.

Sometimes the *left hemisphere person* is unable to decide whether it is winter by simply looking out the window at snow-drifts and leafless trees. He may deduce that it is winter from the fact that the month is January, but the simple visual impression escapes him.

Generally the emotional outlook of these patients is easy going and cheerful, even when they have a pattern of chronic depression or preoccupation with their illness in their normal state. It appears that the left brain is basically optimistic and 'laissez-faire' even when the reality of their situation is depressing.

The right hemisphere person

When a patient receives shock therapy on the left side only, making him temporarily a right hemisphere person, his emotional outlook is transformed in the negative direction and he tends to become more morose and pessimistic about his present situation and future prospects. His speech activity is greatly reduced. He is taciturn, and, instead of answering questions in words, he prefers to respond in mime or gesture. It is difficult to converse with him, as he is inattentive to speech unless it is very loud. He often becomes silent after briefly answering one or two questions.

The speech of the right hemisphere person shows a sharply diminished vocabulary and does not include words for abstract concepts.

He has difficulty recalling names of objects, especially if they are infrequently used, but he is capable of explaining the purpose of any object or showing how it is used. His speech is made up of very simple sentences and often of isolated words. It is necessary to speak to him in very short and simplified sentences to be understood. His intonation and ability to recognise intonation is better than in the normal state.

His hearing for non-verbal sounds is excellent and, in fact, he is more attentive to and better at perceiving natural sounds such as crashing surf than he would be with both halves of his brain working. He recognises music immediately and tends to hum along with it without even being asked.

Apparently the lack of competition from the left brain improves the performance of these tasks.

The task of matching geometric shapes covered with confusing colours and shapes is no problem to the right hemisphere person.

Spotting missing details on pictures and memorising complex shapes is likewise easy. While he cannot say where he is or even give a date or year, he is visually oriented and is able to observe that he is in a hospital, without knowing which one. He recognises the consulting room where he is sitting, although he cannot explain its purpose. He can look out of the window and determine what the season is, though he does not know the date.

If a right hemisphere person is asked to arrange in pairs four cards with 'V', '5', '10', and 'X' on them, he will match them by visual appearance (5 with 10, V with X) rather than by abstract numeric value.

A left hemisphere person will do just the opposite and match numeric values (V with 5, 10 with X). A normal person would probably notice that there are two ways to match them and ask which strategy is desired.

Both the right and left hemisphere seem to have their own unique but overlapping archives of knowledge. While the right hemisphere person does not *know* many of the words and abstract concepts that the left hemisphere person does, he has his own unique store of visual memories, which the left hemisphere does not *know*.

Vadim Deglin agrees with Roger Sperry that we are indeed two separate conscious entities in the same bony cranium.

Let us now combine the neurology of MacLean's triune brain with the functional lateralization of the two cerebral hemispheres and trace an external stimulus from origin to perception (see Figure 2.9).

Anatomically, the whole brain within the skull is made up of two, almost identical halves. Each half has the same triune structure and each of these structures is connected to its fellow structure on the other side by an inter-communicating band of nerve fibres. The two reptilian brains are connected by fibres making up the anterior commissure; the two paleomammalian brains (limbic systems) by the hippocampal commissure; and the neomammalian brains (neocortices) by the corpus callosum.

Naturally, each individual half has its own intrahemispheric communicating fibres – that is, left reptilian-paleomammalian-neomammalian connections – and the right has similar connections.

Let us take an initial stimulus such as a pinprick to the right hand. We know that in the majority of cases it would result in an immediate withdrawal of the right hand from the pin itself. This primary reaction would be of a reflex nature originating in the spinal cord and not involving the central nervous system. The latter would be brought into action to determine how to avoid another prick by the same pin, and might involve complicated avoidance manoeuvres involving cortical decisions.

If we take another initial stimulus, such as a single cry from a baby, the cry would be received as an auditory stimulus and would

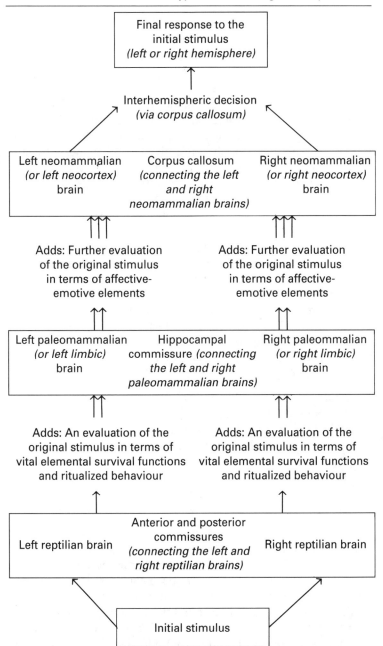

Figure 2.9 Course of an external stimulus in the cerebral hemispheres

probably not involve any reflex action but nevertheless produce a very prompt reaction from an anxious mother or father; the reaction would have originated from the cortical decision of their two hemispheres.

If we ignore reflex responses, we can say that the neurological pathways to the cortex from all initial stimuli are similar and involve genetic and learned (experience) patterns of behaviour which modify the eventual cortical response. For example, in Figure 2.9, an initial stimulus is received simultaneously by both left and right reptilian brains and is analysed and interpreted by them. Clothed with this evaluation, the stimulus is passed on to the two paleomammalian (limbic) brains.

This evaluation of the initial stimulus is in terms of elementary functions vital for survival.

Receiving this now modified stimulus, the two paleomammalian brains further add to its evaluation with affective and emotive elements before passing it on, in turn, to the two neomammalian (neocortices) brains.

Both cerebral hemispheres now, for the first time, have knowledge of an initial external stimulus affecting the body. In addition, the stimulus is accompanied by primitive interpretations which will help the neocortices in their final evaluation.

The sequence of events in the cerebral hemispheres is now:

1 evaluation of the modified stimulus by both hemispheres;
2 interhemispheric decision, via the corpus callosum, as to which hemisphere feels it is better suited for the task;
3 the chosen hemisphere now takes over as the dominant hemisphere in this particular task, inhibiting those functions of the non-selected hemisphere it does not require – it does this by activation of the reticular formation;
4 response to the stimulus by the task-specific hemisphere.

To summarize: the functional anatomy of the brain has been described in terms of P.D. MacLean's triune brain along with its ability to lateralize specific tasks to one hemisphere or the other. These asymmetrical functions have been considered in the light of Sperry and his co-workers' research on split-brained patients. As a result, it has been possible to build up a character assessment of both the left and right hemispheres which has been supported to quite a large degree by the findings of Vadim Deglin using unilateral ECT.

In the last few years, research workers in the field of hemispheric asymmetry have mapped out many more detailed functions in the brain specific to each hemisphere. Knowledge of this subject is now very extensive and increasing rapidly. Apart from the many papers published in the various scientific journals, several books are now available, such as: *The Right Hemisphere* (Ardila and Ostrosky-Solis 1984);[28] *The Dual Brain* (Benson and Zaidel 1985);[29] *Duality and Unity of the Brain* (Ottoson 1987);[30] *Cerebral Lateralization* (Geschwind and Galaburda 1987);[31] and others.

Although the majority of this research has nothing to do with hypnosis, it is possible to relate the various character/functions of the right hemisphere to those of a hypnotized person and find a remarkable similarity.

We can now postulate the following. *Because a person in an hypnotic state, particularly a deep somnambulistic state, exhibits the same cognitive and behavioural functions now attributed by neurological research to the right hemisphere, then it would suggest that the state of hypnosis is right hemisphere-orientated.*

We can also postulate that the mechanism of going into an hypnotic state involves either a shift into right hemisphere function, or an inhibition of the left hemisphere, or both.

Entering into an hypnotic state by inhibition of the left hemisphere offers some advantages over other theoretical mechanisms. As already mentioned, there is a perfectly good, built-in, neurophysiological mechanism available in the brain to effect this inhibition; namely, the inhibitory fibres of the reticular formation (Wyke 1960).[32]

Then again, in the hypnotic state varying depths are recorded, the deepest of which is the so-called *somnambule state*. If hypnosis is achieved by inhibition of the left hemisphere, then the degree of inhibition of this hemisphere would account for the variation of depths; a light trance state would involve only a partial inhibition, whereas the extreme somnambule depth would correspond to a much greater degree of inhibition.

The hypothesis put forward is as follows: *that when we hypnotize an individual we alter his state of consciousness and that this altered state of consciousness is very similar indeed to that of a patient known to be working in a right hemisphere mode.*

Support for this theory is discussed in the next chapter.

Chapter 3

Evidence for the hypnotic state as a right hemisphere-orientated task
A critical review

Some of the evidence presented is based on observation and must be judged accordingly, the rest is based on the results obtained from experiments involving the use of hypnosis. Together they add up sufficiently for serious consideration to be given to this theory.

TIME DISTORTION

Zimbardo et al. (1972)[1] found that subjects given time distortion instructions under hypnosis were able to experience a change in time awareness.

Bramwell (1921)[2] showed that subjects under hypnosis who were given a post-hypnotic instruction to perform a certain task at a later *specific* time (when out of hypnosis), were able to do so with uncanny accuracy.

It is well recognized that, without being given suggestions relating in any way to time, individuals in the state of hypnosis nevertheless seem to lose the sense of the passage of time. Patients coming out of hypnosis are often surprised to discover how much time has elapsed during the course of treatment. It appears to them that time has stood still; they expected the time when they came out of hypnosis to be almost the same as the time they went into it.

Is there a neurological explanation for these clinical observations? I believe there is, if considered in hemispheric terms.

Disorders of time appreciation can, according to Cutting (1990),[3] be summarized as follows:

1 abnormal tempo to events;
2 incorrect ordering of events;

3 disordered sense of duration of past events;
4 disordered sense of the passage of time.

Cutting goes on to state that, despite the paucity of reports available, what evidence is at hand would suggest that where disorders of time appreciation occur, right hemisphere damage, or dysfunction, is the cause.

This implies that the right hemisphere is the regulatory factor where time appreciation is concerned, and would therefore account for the ability of the hypnotist to manipulate this function if, under hypnosis, the patient is working in a right hemisphere mode.

However, it is interesting to consider the results of Efron's (1963)[4] experiments, which led him to suggest that areas in the left hemisphere (the temporal lobe) are concerned with temporal discrimination. Cutting,[5] in explaining Efron's findings, pointed out that the methods he used depended on the brain making a categorical decision. The left hemisphere can categorize, and those disorders where spatial and temporal analysis can be carried out using categorical means could arise through left hemisphere dysfunction.

It seems to me that where 'the sense of passage of time' is concerned (Cutting's fourth element), the sequential (mathematical) procession of time units (first, second, third, fourth and so on) categorized as a linear progression is ideally suited to the left hemisphere, and it is the left hemisphere that should get the job!

If the time-appreciation regulatory factor is a function of the right hemisphere, then in the normal waking state the right hemisphere would *instruct* the left hemisphere to, as it were, start the clock – keep the time.

Under hypnosis, left hemisphere function is inhibited and this 'chronological' factor repressed, which would explain 'time standing still'. It would also explain how chronological instructions given under hypnosis could be carried out in the waking state by the right hemisphere instructing the left.

THE VERBAL DESCRIPTIVE FACTOR

The verbal descriptive factor is a property of the left hemisphere, and the right hemisphere has to rely on the left hemisphere for a *verbal* description of an object.

If, under hypnosis, the subject is shown an object such as a pencil and told that this is a 'ruler', then asked to pick out a ruler from a group of objects (including a ruler) he will pick out a pencil.

Under hypnosis the subject has inhibited the left hemisphere's verbally descriptive function by the induction method of the hypnotist and has substituted the hypnotist's verbally descriptive function. So if the hypnotist verbally suggests that an object of a certain shape is verbally represented by the word 'ruler', the right hemisphere must accept it verbatim. This could explain not only the therapeutic value of hypnosis in certain conditions but also one of its dangers. If it is indeed correct that a subject in hypnosis has inhibited his or her own left hemisphere and has substituted his or her verbal influence by that of the hypnotist, then he or she could be emotionally manipulated by the words of the hypnotist. In the waking state the subject's left hemisphere would merely supply the verbal label for an object and leave the emotional content to be supplied by the right hemisphere. Under hypnosis, however, the word could be delivered with an emotional content already placed there by the hypnotist's right hemisphere. This substituted emotional content need not necessarily be the same as that normally used by the subject's own right hemisphere. For instance, the word 'spider' produces an emotional tag of horror in a spider-phobic subject. By using the word 'spider' under hypnosis with a calm, pleasant and reassuring emotional surround, then one could expect a re-educative effect. On the other hand, another name – say, a personal surname – could be associated with an extreme feeling of anxiety the opposite of which the subject would normally feel. This manipulation could prove undesirable.

DREAMS

Some evidence suggests that dreams and dreaming are primarily right hemisphere functions. Damage to certain areas of the right hemisphere causes cessation of dreaming in patients who previously dreamed normally. These same patients also lose their capacity to visualize when awake (Humphrey and Zangwill 1951).[6]

The American surgeon Wilder Penfield (1959),[7] when operating on epileptic patients, used microelectrodes to stimulate various areas of the cortex in order to pinpoint the exact source of the fits.

Throughout these procedures carried out under local anaesthetic only, the patient was wide awake and in full verbal communication with the surgeon.

When electric currents were applied to the right hemisphere an amazing 'double consciousness' ensued. While the patients were fully aware that they were in the operating theatre talking to the surgeon, they also saw themselves as in a dream in which they were, say, shaking hands with relatives in South Africa! These visual illusions and memory flashbacks associated with the feeling of a double consciousness only occurred when the right hemisphere was stimulated. Stimulation of the left hemisphere merely affected various speech and muscle movements. Normal people never experience this fascinating double consciousness, so it would appear that the electrical stimulus had overcome the inhibitory effect of the reticular formation and made both verbal and nonverbal hemispheres function simultaneously (like having both dip- and main-beam on at the same time).

However, if one considers Freud's belief that dreams are an essential part of problem solving, and correlate this idea with interhemispheric discrepancies as envisaged in cameral analysis, then the left hemisphere must take some part in the dream process. The work of Greenberg and Farah (1986)[8] would suggest just this: they consider that an intact left hemisphere is essential to the dreaming process.

Cohen's hypothesis (1977)[9] went a step further in suggesting that changes in cerebral dominance occur during dream sleep; an initial right hemisphere dominance gradually gives way to a left hemisphere dominance as the dreaming process comes to its end.

Joseph (1988)[10] also agrees with the Freudian problem-solving concept of dreams but considers that all the evidence now available points to their taking place in a fully functional right hemisphere during low-level left hemisphere arousal.

Although more research is needed, it appears that we can reasonably consider dreams to be largely a right hemisphere prerogative, and if, as happens under hypnosis, dreams and hallucinations can be easily conjured up by the hypnotist – for example, 'You are now in South Africa shaking hands with your relatives' – then it seems possible that a subject under hypnosis is working in a right hemisphere mode.

HYPNOTIZABILITY OF THE POPULACE

All scales of hypnotizability (for example, the Stanford Scale of Hypnotic Susceptibility and others), whichever groups are studied, show the following.

A universally high hypnotizability factor in children

Why should this be? It could be argued that children are developing lateralization and that left hemisphere skills are in their infancy. They exist more in a fantasy world, which is a right hemisphere function, and, therefore, are more easily able to slip into this world. However, some interesting work was done in 1981 by Dr Marjorie Hogan (1982)[11] of the Children's Health Center in Minneapolis in which she studied the effect of hypnosis on brain-stem auditory-evoked response in children aged six to eleven. She found that all children, irrespective of whether they were under hypnosis or not, were able to modify their response to auditory stimuli by simple suggestion alone, from which she concluded that children very easily move into an altered state of consciousness with or without formal hypnotic induction, and that this showed a very quick and easy shift into the right hemisphere function.

High hypnotizability of art students, low hypnotizability of science students

Work done by Josephine Hilgard (1970)[12] of Stanford University on students showed that those in the arts faculties had a universally higher hypnotic susceptibility than those of the science faculties. This can be explained by the fact that the arts subjects require a predominantly right hemisphere function and, therefore, students of the arts live to a greater extent in the right hemisphere and indeed are trained into a greater right lateralization of function. On the other hand, because science students are trained into a more linear, logical and unemotional method of thinking, they are more likely to be left-hemisphere-lateralized individuals and may find more difficulty in shifting into the right hemisphere. This would predispose to a low hypnotizability.

Diminution of hypnotizability with age

With age, degenerative processes may slow down the inhibitory mechanism of the reticular formation, and it could be argued that the ageing process diminishes the lability of hemispheric change.

Older people tend to hang on to one mode of function; they become more garrulous and less imaginative; that is, they stick in their left hemisphere mode rather in the same way that their eyesight at the age of forty-five loses its power of accommodation.

Low hypnotizability of schizophrenic patients

It is generally accepted that schizophrenics are very difficult, if not impossible, to hypnotize. In the early stages of the condition they show a degree of resistance but as the disease progresses hypnosis becomes increasingly difficult.

If the hypnotic state depends on the ability of the subject to function in a right hemisphere mode, then any disease causing lateralized dysfunction should, *ipso facto*, affect hypnotizability.

Work on schizophrenia done by Gareth Jones and Julian Miller (1981)[13] indicated that the interhemispheric conduction time across the corpus callosum is effectively zero. This suggests that schizophrenia is a split-brained condition akin to agenesis of the corpus callosum, unrecognized through the use of compensatory ipsilateral pathways.

Unfortunately, this work has not been confirmed, and it may be that methods of measuring the interhemispheric conduction time is not accurate enough to warrant their conclusions. However, work published by Sheppard *et al.* (1983)[14] of the Charing Cross Hospital, using PET scanning, supports the hypothesis that abnormality in hemisphere laterality may underlie schizophrenic illness. Similarly work done by John Gruzelier (1976)[15] in skin conductance experiments on schizophrenic and depressed patients gave support to the lateralized dysfunction model of mental illness and implicated a left hemisphere disorder in schizophrenia.

EYE MOVEMENTS

Individuals rapt in thought can be observed with their eyes looking upwards to the left or the right. M.E. Day (1964),[16] in a paper relating to these eye movements, postulated that in right-handed individuals, if they move their eyes to the left while they are thinking, it would indicate a preference for processing information in the right hemisphere.

In 1969, Bakan,[17] basing his work on this postulate, reported a significant correlation between hypnotic susceptibility and right hemisphere preference. These findings were later supported by Gur and Gur in 1975,[18] when they found that right-handed, left-eye movers scored better than right movers on a hypnotic susceptibility scale. However, this work has been somewhat negated since by Erlichman and Weinberger (1979),[19] who found that there was no evidence to justify the use of lateral eye movements as a method of studying hemispheric function.

On the other hand, in 1979 Graham and Pernicano,[20] in their paper entitled 'Autokinetic effects under hypnosis', showed a significant increase in the apparent left movement of a light source in right-handed individuals under hypnosis (the hypnotic patients were asked to report on the movement of a steady light by tracing the movement on a pad when under hypnosis), and Graham and Pernicano concluded that there was definite evidence of a shift to the right hemisphere mode under hypnosis.

DICHOTIC LISTENING TESTS

Dichotic listening tests are tests in which a subject is delivered a different word to each ear simultaneously by means of headphones separately connected to different word sources. For instance, the word 'dog' is transmitted to the left ear and at the same time a similar word, such as 'cog', is transmitted to the right ear. The subject is asked to write down the word he or she hears. The answers are analysed, and it has been found that words received by the right ear are distinguished more times than those received by the left. This advantage is explained by the right ear having a direct route to the left hemisphere's speech centre, whereas the neural connections of the left ear have the less direct route through the corpus callosum.

Frumkin, in 1978,[21] in a paper entitled 'Changes in cerebral hemispheric lateralisation with hypnosis', produced under normal conditions what one would expect: namely, a right-ear advantage in dichotic listening tests because of left hemisphere dominance of verbal tasks. But he found that under hypnosis this produced a significant reduction in right-ear advantage, suggesting a real reduction in left hemisphere influence, and from this Frumkin suggested that the state of hypnosis was associated with the right hemisphere.

ELECTROENCEPHALOGRAPHY STUDIES

Brain activity can be measured by placing electrodes at various places on the scalp which record, in the form of a graph, electrical discharges that are taking place in the brain. Different activities produce different wave-patterns, labelled as alpha, beta, delta and theta.

At first sight, studies of the electroencephalogram would appear to be the obvious way to see whether, under hypnosis, there is any difference in activity between the two hemispheres, particularly if one could take separate EEGs of the right and left hemispheres simultaneously. It was surprising, therefore, to find that there was very little EEG work done in this field with reference to the separate hemispheres. From 1947 to 1972 no fewer than twenty papers were published concerning EEG readings under hypnosis, in transcendental meditation, autogenic training, and using emotionally significant words. The results were varied and sometimes contradictory.

By 1972, however, what had emerged was that under hypnosis the alpha activity was significantly increased. In 1974, Ullyett et al.,[22] published a paper entitled 'Quantitative EEG analysis during hypnosis', which showed without much doubt that increased alpha activity could be used as a measure of the hypnotic state. But it was not until later that this was used to show that there was a difference in alpha activity between the two hemispheres when the subject was in hypnosis.

Galin and Ornstein (1972),[23] at the University of California Medical Center, recorded EEG alpha signals from the left and right hemispheres simultaneously while the subjects did verbal or spatial tasks, and, rather excitingly, found that the EEG showed that normal people (as opposed to split-brain people) tend to think with one side of the brain or the other: verbal tasks with the left hemisphere, spatial tasks with the right hemisphere. Although these were significant findings they were not related to hypnosis.

MacLeod-Morgan and Lack (1982)[24] did a series of EEG recordings in the waking state on highly hypnotizable people and subjects with a low hypnotizability. They have shown that highly hypnotizable subjects lateralize their brains more specifically for right and left hemisphere-mediated tasks than do low hypnotizability subjects. They conclude that the EEG evidence supports the contentions that hypnosis is a right hemisphere task.

Confirmation of the work of MacLeod-Morgan and Lack has come from Budapest University in Hungary. Istvan Mészáros (1982)[25] studied evoked potential correlates of verbal versus imagery coding in hypnosis. His findings demonstrated shifts in evoked potential amplitude towards the right hemisphere during hypnosis. In a later paper (1986),[26] Mészáros showed that the evidence of both electroencephalographic and behavioural performance studies supported enhanced right hemisphere activation during hypnosis. Crawford et al. (1989)[27] demonstrated a shift towards greater right hemisphere activity during hypnosis of highly hypnotizable individuals.

In considering these EEG studies it must be pointed out that the EEG shows the measurement of only a very small depth of the external surface of the cerebral cortex, and it is impossible to pinpoint the exact site of activity. While it is reasonable to suppose that the cortex itself is in fact the source, it is also possible that the electrical potentials measured at the surface could emanate from much deeper structures, such as the limbic system. Until EEG studies produce more accurate source data, the danger of over-enthusiastic interpretation of their evidence must be resisted. However, world-wide research is occurring in this field and the results are awaited with interest.

HAPTIC PROCESSING TESTS AND ELECTRODERMAL RESPONSES

Experiments have been published (Gruzelier et al. 1984)[28] in which Haptic Processing Tests have been compared on volunteer subjects either in or out of hypnosis. The task involved the discrimination of plastic letters from plastic numbers by feeling the shapes with the hands while blindfolded. Measurements were taken of the sorting times of both the left hand and the right hand separately. Gruzelier et al. (1984)[29] also measured electrodermal responses from both hands in subjects in the normal waking state and then under hypnosis.

The objective of these experiments was to examine the theory that implicates right hemisphere processes (or the reduced involvement of the left hemisphere) in the hypnotic state. Their conclusion was that hypnotically susceptible subjects had a pre-existing left hemisphere bias, and that a prerequisite for successful hypnotic induction was the inhibition of the left hemisphere.

As far as I am concerned, however, there are two other very important factors illustrated by these experiments:

1 They indicated that a shift in lateral cerebral influences occurred in susceptible subjects under hypnosis, and that the evidence was consistent with the view that in hypnosis there is a release of right hemisphere activity.
2 They indicated that people with lability processes in keeping with their cognitive demands are more likely to be hypnotically good subjects.

This, of course, confirms MacLeod-Morgan and Lack's (1982)[30] findings that those individuals who were able to use the correct hemisphere habitually for any given task (for example, left hemisphere for a verbal task and right hemisphere for a spatial task) were not only intelligent but were also hypnotically susceptible subjects.

THE EVIDENCE OF MEMORY

The work of A.R. Luria and E.G. Simernitskaya (1977)[31] of Moscow University has shown that the human memory system consists of two separate cognitive functions: namely, *intentional memory* – that is, the intentional learning of, say, a part in a play; and *involuntary memory*, where, without any conscious effort, ordinary events of everday life are capable of recall if necessary. They have also shown that intentional memory is a left hemisphere function but involuntary memory is a function of the right hemisphere.

As is well known, memory recall under hypnosis is often quite dramatic, and involves the recall of material when absolutely no effort was being made by the person to memorize it (Reiff and Scheerer 1959),[32] as, for instance, the events or presents one received on one's fifth birthday (Erickson 1965).[33] Whether this material is an absolutely true memory of past events, or whether it contains distinct elements of fantasy matters little from the thera-peutic point of view. What does matter is the strength and charac-ter of the repressed (or forgotten) emotional content associated with the event and the act of recalling and re-living it under hypnosis (Freud and Breuer 1895).[34] However, the very fact that we can, to some extent, enhance this involuntary form of memory under hypnosis implicates the right hemisphere.

THE HIDDEN OBSERVER PHENOMENON (HILGARD AND HILGARD 1989)[35]

In 1977 Ernest and Josephine Hilgard induced an hypnotic deafness in a subject, who, as a result, did not respond to questions or loud noises. However, when the subject was asked whether there was any part of him that was aware of the noises, to the astonishment of the Hilgards he replied in the affirmative. The Hilgards attributed this phenomenon to the presence of what they term a *hidden observer*.

Similar results have been obtained with subjects in whom the sensation of pain has been hypnotically reduced. These subjects show no reaction to painful stimuli and may even verbally deny the feeling of pain, but at the same time they can respond by tracing onto paper an accurate graph of changes in the pain gradient with a pen in their right hand.

This apparent paradox of awareness in hypnotized subjects can be explained in terms of left hemisphere inhibition (or suppression), and indeed this has been experimentally verified.

One of Sperry's team (Gazzaniga 1972)[36] using the Wada technique knocked out the left hemisphere of a patient by injecting sodium amytal into the patient's left carotid artery. In the few minutes during which the *left* hemisphere was temporarily suppressed an object was placed in the *left* hand of the patient but totally obscured from the patient's view. When the sodium amytal effect had worn off the patient *verbally* denied any knowledge of any object whatsoever but was able to identify the object accurately by *pointing* to it among a pile of different objects!

In discussing this experiment by Gazzaniga, Frumkin (1978)[37] states: 'The split in consciousness by the contrasting verbal and non-verbal reports from the amytal patients clearly results from a change in cerebral lateralisation, namely temporary supression of left hemisphere dominance.'

The finding that hypnosis temporarily reduces left hemisphere dominance strongly suggests a cerebral lateralization explanation for the hypnotically produced split in consciousness noted by Hilgard, the 'hidden observer' being the suppressed left hemisphere.

Memory and the *hidden observer* evidence come together interestingly in a case published by Professor Martin Orne (1951)[38] and quoted again in his address to the Fourth European Congress in Hypnosis and Psychosomatic Medicine held in Oxford in 1987. In this paper Professor Orne was considering the validity of age regression under hypnosis and the truthfulness of its memory recall, and quoted an adult patient of his whom he regressed back to the age of six. Under hypnosis, at the apparently regressed age of six, the patient was asked to draw a tree, a person, a wigwam (tepee) and a house. These drawings were then compared with drawings of the same subjects that the patient had drawn himself when he was actually at the age of six and which had been saved by his parents. The similarity was really quite remarkable and, had there been no comparisons available, investigators would have accepted the drawings made under hypnosis as a positive example of age regression. However, each one of the drawings made under hypnosis showed slight differences of a more sophisticated nature than the originals. For instance, the tree had more generalized leaves, whereas in the original each leaf had been separately drawn. The person had two ears and a nose; these were absent in the original. The wigwam had four tent-poles sticking out of the peak; the original was just a triangular-shaped object. And the house had a wall and a path, giving an almost three-dimensional effect, which was lacking in the original. Professor Orne considered that these differences showed that hypnosis did not produce *true* age regression. He maintained that had it done so, in no way could the more sophisticated embellishments have crept in. But there could be another explanation.

It could be argued that the age regression under hypnosis was taking place in the right hemisphere and was probably as true a regression to that age as was possible, but it was the left hemisphere's influence which was responsible for the more sophisticated components in the sketches. Furthermore, in the light of the right hemisphere theory I would expect some interference from the non-regressed left hemisphere in keeping with the *hidden observer* effect.

As more research is done on hemispheric lateralization, more and more cognitive functions are found to be the prerogative of either the right or the left cerebral hemisphere. It is also becoming more and more obvious that the human brain functions asymmetrically. These neurological discoveries have profound psychological implications, so much so that old theories on the origin of the neuroses and psychoses must be re-examined and their treatment reviewed. The most important of these new concepts of significance to hypnosis are the following four.

1 Hemispheric specialization

Zaidel, in 1985,[39] and Bogen, in 1987,[40] have been able to show that there are two separate principles underlying hemispheric functions. The first is hemispheric specialization, and it covers a wide range of tasks.

At one end are those tasks that can be performed equally well by both hemispheres, although each hemisphere uses a totally different processing method to produce the same result. At the other end are those tasks totally specific to one specialized hemisphere; for example, the phonological analysis of the printed word is entirely task-specific to the left hemisphere.

2 Hemispheric independence

Split-brain experiments have shown that both hemispheres are conscious entities in themselves, as indeed did investigation of brain-damaged individuals who were known to have one hemisphere destroyed and yet were conscious and could carry out relatively normal and meaningful lives.

Critics, however, were quick to point out that, as these were damaged brains, their very abnormality might account for the research findings. But as research continues in this field it is becoming more obvious that independent functioning of the two hemispheres is the norm rather than the exception in ordinary individuals.[41]

The fact that it can be shown that there are task-specific functions which are the sole responsibility of one hemisphere must support the concept of hemispheric independence at work in ordinary individuals. *If this is so, then we have here a source of potential interhemispheric conflict.*

3 Hemispheric dissociation

To give an example, an experiment was carried out on a split-brain patient in which non-emotional geometric shapes were randomly presented to both hemispheres by means of a tachistoscope.[42] In the midst of these shapes a photograph of a nude figure was shown to the right hemisphere only. The subject reacted by giggling and blushing but was never able to explain this behaviour verbally. This concept is important to clinical psychiatry in that it provides a neurological basis for the empirical idea that repressed material is contained in a mental compartment inaccessible to verbal contact and, furthermore, can affect the autonomic nervous system. It also illustrates how the right hemisphere draws attention to a *surprise anomaly* by the use of body-language, and that the autonomic nervous system is part and parcel of this communication system (blushing).

4 Interhemispheric antagonism

Jerre Levy (1972),[43] working with split-brained patients, showed that the two disconnected hemispheres *working on the same task* process *the same* sensory information in distinctly different ways: namely, temporal analysis for the left, and spatial synthesis for the right.

The method of processing information by temporal analysis involves an analytic approach in a linear and syllogistic mode for which words are an ideal medium; spatial synthesis, on the other hand, solves problems by involving multiple convergent determinants giving a holistic and emotional overview which is ideally suitable for music or spatial relations. By these means the brain has the tremendous advantage of being able to tackle the same problem from two different angles and thus doubles the chances of its being solved. For instance, one can navigate a boat mathematically by using a compass, charts, a clock, and by measuring the speed of the vessel; this way would make use of the left hemisphere. On the other hand, one could use the spatial capabilities of the right hemisphere by lining up various features of the landscape or the stars with the prow, sides or stern of the boat. Furthermore, one method can be used to check the results of the other, or to help it, or both, or they can be used independently if required.

However, there is a disadvantage.

Jerre Levy (1970)[44] has made the very important observation that the two hemispheres, working on the same task and with the same sensory input, can interpret the same information to reach different and *conflicting* conclusions, and the result of this mutual antagonism shows up as a behavioural disturbance. The importance of these two factors is in the realization that the human mind has two distinct ways of looking at, and interpreting, a *single* event.

To the left hemisphere the logical and unemotional evaluation of an incident could, to the right hemisphere, be an emotional catastrophe causing deep-seated fear and anxiety, but, because of the verbal dominance of the left hemisphere it is often only the left hemisphere's evaluation that is communicated in, say, a doctor/patient interview.

In Chapter 2 I gave as an example an incident in a television programme in which Professor F. Frankel hypnotized a volunteer and regressed her back to a happy event in her childhood. Unfortunately this 'verbally' (left hemisphere) happy event turned out to be an 'emotionally' (right hemisphere) catastrophic occasion, and the hypnotized patient ended up in tears. *A therapeutic advantage can, and must, be taken of being able to separate this emotional dichotomy by the use of hypnosis, and we must persistently search in our patient's past for such events.*

In Chapter 4 I discuss the role of hypnosis in this new psychological environment, and suggest *cameral analysis* as a method of treatment which makes use of the right hemisphere mediation of the hypnotic phenomenon. Cameral analysis also recognizes the possibility of problems arising from hemispheric asymmetry.

Part II

Practical applications

Twin brethren dwell within me, twins of strife,
And either fights to free him from the other;
One grips the earth in savage lust of life,
Clutches the ground and wallows in the mire;
The other lifts himself and struggles free,
Tearing the chain that binds him to his brother,
Beating the air with wings of vast desire
Toward the far realm of his great ancestry.
Goethe, Faust, 11, 1112–1117

Chapter 4

Cameral analysis

Many fields of medical research tend to be so compartmentalized that their disciplines remain separate. Although neurology and psychology have developed extensively, it is only recently that the two research fields have come together in the new science of neuropsychology. Despite this development, few are relating the hypnotic phenomenon to these new concepts, particularly in the practical – that is, the therapeutical – field.

I have tried to fill in this void.

What follows is a description of my method, cameral analysis, which utilizes these new concepts in clinical practice. Although some of the techniques are well known to psychotherapy, there is a distinct difference in how they are applied.

Theoretically the left hemisphere's *modus operandi* is by means of 'temporal analysis', and is unencumbered by emotional interference. Temporal analysis has distinct communicative limitations; it is frequently impossible to express, in terms of temporal analysis, a solution derived by 'spatial synthesis' (the *modus operandi* of the right hemisphere), and, of course, vice versa. Furthermore, the right hemisphere has to incorporate into its solution the often illogicality of emotion.

This can lead to discrepancies between the two hemispheres.

In my opinion, the origins of a neurosis can lie in interhemispheric discrepancies.

These discrepancies can take three forms.

Direct conflicts: Where emotional desires favouring one course of action are in direct disagreement with another deduced logically.

The conflict arises out of this possibility of holding different interpretations of the same incoming stimulus. Naturally, in the majority of interpretations, the conclusions reached are the same, or sufficiently similar to avoid any conflict. Where, however, conflict does occur, evidence shows[1] that only one of the interpretations will be tolerated, which, *ipso facto*, means the other has to be repressed in order for the body as a whole to react to the stimulus.

The use of repression in this way may result in a satisfactory conclusion, particularly if the stimulus was a minor one and the eventual outcome was of no particular significance. If, however, the decision involved a vital, long-term, emotional overtone, repression would also continue long-term and demand a great deal of mental energy to sustain. Under these circumstances it is often difficult to maintain a complete repression, and this may result in the surfacing of symptoms indicating the conflict.

Split-brained patients exhibit this conflict in a very direct way. For instance, a patient found her left hand fighting her right hand in the choice of clothes to wear on a cold day. The right hand (left hemisphere) favoured a logical, warm tweed, whereas the left hand tried to impose a more attractive but less practical dress.

Differences in interpretation: These are not necessarily conflicting, but may offer two differing interpretations of the same event. For instance, a child may *logically* accept punishment for a misdemeanour but *emotionally* conclude that 'Mummy does not love me any more'; for example, the child who has been repeatedly told never to play with a ball in the hallway of his home in case he breaks a valuable antique vase standing there, and furthermore, were this to happen, that he would be severely punished. When it did happen, the child logically accepted his punishment but emotionally could only interpret hate in his mother's face. The result was the basis of a gradually developing anxiety state relieved many years later by abreaction of the event.

Another example is Professor Frankel's volunteer (see Chapter 2, p. 40) who, when asked under hypnosis to go back to a happy event in her childhood, ended up with a very different and unhappy interpretation of the event.

Differences in knowledge: One hemisphere may be aware of certain facts not directly available to the other. This possibility was dramatically shown in the experiment carried out by Gazzaniga (1972)[2] and quoted in Chapter 3 in explanation of the 'hidden observer' phenomenon. As previously mentioned, Gazzaniga used the Wada technique to knock out the left hemisphere of a normal individual volunteer. In the few minutes during which the left hemisphere was temporarily suppressed, an object was placed in the *left* hand of the patient but totally obscured from the patient's view. When the sodium amytal effect had worn off the patient *verbally* denied any knowledge of any object being placed in his hand but was able to identify the object accurately by *pointing* to it among a pile of different objects!

If this is so, and the source of neurotic symptoms emanates from the clash of discordant interpretations of the same sensory input by the two hemispheres, then in order successfully to treat such symptoms the therapist must first of all:

1 understand *both* interpretations, and then
2 resolve the conflict by measures which are both understandable and acceptable to each hemisphere.

Cameral analysis is designed to do just this.

Cameral analysis is what it implies, namely, single chamber analysis ('camera' = domed chamber) in which the left and right chambers (hemispheres) are interviewed (analysed) in two separate modes and in two separate states of consciousness.

Mode one: analysis of the left hemisphere whereby the therapist questions in depth the left hemisphere's interpretation of the presenting problem. In other words, one takes the usual medical and psychiatric history by verbal questioning of the patient.

It is particularly important at the same time to observe any body-language the patient communicates and to make notes of it and its context *at the point at which it occurred*. Such signs as, for instance, sighing, blushing, hand-to-face movements, finger tapping, head movements and so on often draw attention to, or negate, statements made verbally.

Dr Dabney Ewin tells of a patient of his who, when asked the question 'Do you love your husband?' answered verbally, 'Of course I do!' while at the same time shaking her head from side to side!

The second mode is that of the right hemisphere. This involves first, questioning the right hemisphere with the patient in hypnosis; secondly, regressing the patient under hypnosis to incidents concerning his or her problem and opening up details in the patient's *involuntary memory* store; thirdly, encouraging the abreaction of relevant events under hypnosis, thus allowing the patient to re-live the event at a much more mature period in their life when they are able to cope with the situation, rather than having to repress it, as previously, in order to achieve mental stability. (Shell-shock is an extreme example of this where the memory of the incident may include the inevitability of death. By abreacting the incident in what is now a survival situation, the patient releases the horror of the emotional memory and begins logically to accept their survival as being the true fact.) Fourthly, use is made of *re-educative symptom exposure* techniques while the patient is under hypnosis to change the emotional complexion of an event (past, present or on-going) into a more acceptable interpretation involving less fear, anxiety, anger, frustration and so forth.

These right hemisphere techniques utilize music, poetry, song, dance, fantasy, guided imagery, transitional objects, dreams or writing. For example, with the patient under hypnosis, I may use a Chopin nocturne to accompany ego-strengthening suggestions, or I may play a piece of recorded music (or a song) of emotional significance to the patient to assist the recall of involuntary memory or life crises. Verbal suggestions are much more powerful if accompanied by music; one sung hymn with very simple words puts over a religious message more powerfully and permanently than a hundred sermons from the pulpit!

Similarly, under hypnosis, if one wants to re-arrange the right hemisphere's interpretation of an event, *use the language of the right hemisphere* – give the message in a holistic, Gestalt form as in a parable; the right hemisphere understands parables and this is why they have a much greater emotional impact.

Again, with the patient under hypnosis, I will choose a poem with a metaphoric content the same as, or similar to, the suggestion I wish to convey, then read it to the patient making sure that they understand how it relates to themselves. They do not necessarily relate verbally, but more with the metaphoric and prosodic comprehension of the right hemisphere.

Prosody,[3] the melodic contour of speech, is responsible for modulating the grammar and semantics of the spoken word and as a result introduces the subtle meanings and emphasis values so important in the understanding of language. Prosody has been shown to be a right hemisphere contribution to language[4] and plays a prime role in poetic impact.

Poetry is a very important factor in the concept of cameral analysis. Some patients write poetry, and if they do, then this is an added bonus; their poems are often more informative than their dreams.

I actually encourage patients, in their leisure hours, to write poetry *on the theme of their problem*, because, in my opinion, poetry is the most powerful way of combining both hemispheres into co-operating in a single task and helps in their mutual understanding of the problem.

Throughout history poems have been used to help the poet overcome periods of stress and anxiety of a personal and public nature: the classic 'lover's lament' helps to reduce the abject despair of the rejected suitor; the pictorial image of England in Robert Browning's 'Home Thoughts from Abroad' helped him overcome his homesickness. There are endless examples.

Most of the techniques used in cameral analysis are well known in psychotherapy; the difference lies in their interpretation in right and left hemisphere function and, of course, the eventual use of this knowledge in helping the two hemispheres to come to terms with each other. Cameral analysis incorporates this interpretation of brain-function into a workable therapeutic method capable of treating the psychoneuroses in a comparatively quick, efficient and effective manner.

This introduction to cameral analysis has so far illustrated its basic principles and outlined its method, but before taking a more detailed look at some of its techniques I would like to draw attention to (1) important differences from psychoanalysis, and (2) apparent anomalies to research findings in neurophysiology.

Cameral analysis involves a very dynamic, interactive approach to the patient as opposed to that of psychoanalysis, which employs more laid-back, passive methods. It is often argued that there are possible dangers in this active approach in so far as the analyst's own character, along with any unresolved problems, will impinge on that of the patient. The result could be a clouded assessment of the patient's problems, which could lead to possible case mismanagement.

The psychoanalytical school places great emphasis on this possible danger and insists on its therapists undergoing an analysis themselves before launching into patient treatment. This to me is an old chestnut and can be applied, in effect, to any psychotherapy. All members of the medical profession, from GPs to consultants, are regularly 'analysing' their patients, particularly if there is a psychological element to their patients' somatic problem.

This, of course, does not deny the argument; it certainly exists, but I think its dangers are very much over-emphasized.

Professor Anthony Clare and other psychiatrists, such as Michael Shepherd and Ernest Gellner,[5,6] have been taking a more detailed look at psychoanalysis and have been disturbed by their findings, a very minor one of which is this insistence on the analysis of future therapists. If one can assume that most therapists are already reasonably well adjusted, then analysis is probably unnecessary, and, of course, it could have a potentially negative effect on their character ('It is like taking the bubbles out of champagne!' as a colleague has remarked). This, along with the cost of psychoanalytical treatment, its never-ending time consumption, and its dubious results, add up to a very negative re-appraisal.

In my opinion the so-called 'talking cure' relies on the left verbal hemisphere for every interpretation of behaviour; even *free association* is 'explained' in verbal terms through the left hemisphere and must be influenced by this hemisphere. The ability of psychoanalysis to get at the direct opinions of right hemisphere thought-processes, apart from dreams, is limited and therefore its knowledge of the true emotional content and its influence on behaviour must be jeopardized. Feedback is clouded by left hemisphere interference, and this itself would contribute to the length of treatment. To me, Freud's mistake was to reject the use of hypnosis in the treatment method he was formulating; in so doing he, in effect, approached the neuroses with one hand (left!) tied behind his back.

Furthermore, the intelligence of patients, their educational background and achievements, as well as their ability to comprehend themselves (that is, the degree of personal insight they can attain) vary enormously.

Psychoanalysis, by insisting that its object is to help patients to understand themselves, narrows its field of influence to those patients who are educated and intelligent enough to get somewhere near this impossible goal. When they do eventually achieve this degree of insight, psychoanalysis does not guarantee an improvement in their condition, which may, in fact, turn out to be worse than their original state. Freud himself made the point that the best one can expect from psychoanalysis is to exchange the misery of neurotic behaviour for ordinary human misery.

Cameral analysis recognizes not only the wide variations in the ability of patients to achieve insight but also in the equally wide variations in their behavioural norm. The aim of cameral analysis is to help the patients back into *their particular* society. This does not necessarily mean that the patients will eventually understand themselves or even, for that matter, their problem. What it does mean is that patients are asked to take a new look at their problems and to re-structure them in such a way as to make them acceptable *within the range of their own personal insight*, however wide or narrow this may be. Cameral analysis could therefore be described as a re-educative, reconstructing and sometimes conciliatory process, taking place between the left (logical) and right (emotional) hemispheres.

The second potential criticism of cameral analysis must come from the excellent research that has been done, and is continuing to be done, on the neurophysiology and biochemistry of the septo-hippocampal system (MacLean's paleomammalian brain, or the limbic system). The vast sums of money that have been poured into this field of research by wealthy drug companies has, for them, paid off handsomely in the development of expensive mood-interfering drugs in the form of the diazepines and monoamine-oxidase inhibitors. Consultant psychiatrist Peter Tyler, writing in the *British Journal of Psychiatry* (1991),[7] states:

Serotonin, or 5-hydroxytryptamine (5-HT), is rapidly becoming as important to biological psychiatry as DNA is to molecular biology. Time after time, investigations into the mechanisms lying behind psychiatric disorders lead back to the 5-HT receptors. This is both encouraging and puzzling. It is encouraging because we now have many drugs available that act on 5-HT receptors, both as agonists and antagonists, and so it seems likely through these, we will be able to improve our treatment of many types of psychiatric disorder. *It is puzzling because the imagination is stretched to believe that the 5-HT receptor is at the heart of psychopathology; some of the changes found are likely to be secondary phenomena and the prime target for investigation likely to lie elsewhere.*

Professor J.A. Gray, in his book *The Neuropsychology of Anxiety* (1982),[8] puts forward his theory that the limbic system is a comparator system in which *expected events* are compared with *actual events*. If there is a mismatch between these two the response is an *anxiety state*.

This to me is extremely interesting in that this is exactly the mechanism I consider to be the cause of a neurosis, anxiety or otherwise, but with one important difference. Instead of the cause of an anxiety neurosis being a mismatch in the limbic system, I lay the blame on *interhemispheric conflict (mismatch)*.

This does not go against Professor Gray's theory in any way if he considers the function of the limbic system to be that of a comparator and not a decision-maker. The comparator, like a good civil servant, assembles the facts, points out the discrepancies, and passes the information on to higher centres for a decision on future action. It is, in fact, a valuable and integral part of the learning process and as such a vital survival mechanism.

In the majority of cases the limbic 'comparisons' are within an acceptable matching range. When a mismatch is reported, the anxiety evoked induces a counteracting hemispheric response, the successful result being stored in the appropriate memory bank. Where counteraction is unsuccessful and continues to remain an insoluble problem, then a permanent state of anxiety will exist. This may be a mild state of anxiety offering little disruption to everyday life; for instance, an aunt of mine who hated travelling would arrive at the station hours before her train was due to make sure she would be in time to catch it. In every other way she was a charming individual who led a very normal life. On the other hand, the quality of life of the claustrophobic recluse is quite unacceptable and demands treatment. In the latter case, if drugs are used, they act by interfering with the comparator process and thus denying the neocortical hemispheres the correct information. No information, or diminished or distorted information, lessens the conflict, and may result in a noticeable improvement in the patient's condition.

Sadly, this is rather like brushing the crumbs under the carpet and, in the case of the psychoneuroses, does not get at the source of the mismatch (discrepancies) of expected and actual events. Furthermore, if the source of the anxiety remains and the drug treatment continues, drug-addiction may complicate the picture and hamper other forms of treatment.

There are thousands of patients in this world who ideally should be lying on a psychiatrist's couch. Unfortunately, they cannot afford the luxury of such treament and will have to be content with drugs. This fact does not lessen the dangers of present drug treatment but calls for further research into more suitable, less addictive drugs, and serves as a good excuse for continuing their use in the treatment of the psychoneuroses.

This argument does not apply, of course, to the psychoses, where drug treatment is of inestimable value and, more often than not, the treatment of choice. In these cases the improvement in their quality of life far outweighs any dangers inherent in the drug treatment, and to many of them has meant an almost complete rehabilitation into the norm of society, something unheard of only a few years ago.

I have tried to point out that, although it is possible to show experimentally that anxiety depends on the activity of the septo-hippocampal system, and that drugs acting at this level can diminish anxiety, it does not follow that we must blame the paleomammalian brain for the cause of an anxiety neurosis and the symptoms it exhibits. My argument is this:

First, consciousness is an essential factor in any neurosis.

A neurotic individual may behave in a peculiar way under certain conditions (e.g., getting into a lift) but otherwise he would appear to be conscious, awake, and capable of looking after himself or herself.

Secondly, we know that neurologically an essential part of consciousness is the presence of *one*, at least, intact hemisphere. This consists of an intact reptilian section, an intact limbic section and an intact neocortex. (From experience of damaged brains due to accidents, injuries, tumours, strokes, and so on, and the occasional child born with an agenesis of one half of the brain – that is, one complete hemisphere – apart from severe mobility problems it is possible to live a conscious, meaningful life as long as one hemisphere is intact.)

Thirdly, the final common path of behaviour that proves us actually to be conscious is through the motor and sensory cortex. *It is not through the limbic system.*

So, although it may well be that anxiety states are generated in the limbic system, or other lower centre for that matter, it is the final path, the neocortex, that is essential in order for them to be expressed.

Without the neocortex there would be no consciousness.

Without consciousness a neurosis could not achieve expression.

To be able to treat a patient, conscious expression is essential.

Therefore, any therapeutic method, *not involving the use of drugs or surgery*, must work through the cortices (cerebral hemispheres).

It follows that any methods that analyse the cortices would be expected to have a therapeutic value, but, as in cameral analysis, if each were analysed separately and with least interference from the other, this method should have a distinct advantage.

I feel it does, and I have found its use rewarding.

Having discussed two possible criticisms of cameral analysis let us examine the method in more detail.

PATIENT'S RECORDS

It is customary in the medical profession to jot down salient features of the patient's medical history as it is recounted. Apart from jogging the memory when writing a return letter to the referring doctor, these notes serve as a recorded history for future reference and follow the patient throughout their life in so-called confidential NHS documents.

Making notes offers no problems where obvious illnesses such as measles, mumps and so forth are concerned. Similarly, operations with no social stigma such as an appendectomy or even a gastrectomy can be recorded in detail. But how confidential are these notes and where does one draw the line?

In my opinion it is the patient's prerogative to decide if he or she wishes certain facts about their lives to be set down in black and white. I take the view that the patient knows he has, for instance, syphilis, that the disease has been thoroughly explained to him, and that were he to become ill in the future it would be of vital importance to his treatment that the doctor in charge of his case should know this fact. Under these circumstances it would be to the benefit of the patient himself for him to inform the doctor. On the other hand, syphilis is curable. It would be unfortunate if some isolated episode occurring in youth could jeopardize his promotion to a responsible job much later in his life just because his NHS notes were in the hands of a Civil Service doctor. Similarly, abortion is by no means universally accepted and it may be to the considerable detriment of the patient for it to be recorded.

On the whole, the great majority of doctors maintain a strict order of confidentiality in accordance with their Hippocratic oath, but their typists take no such oath, although, to be fair, most practices include a clause on confidentiality in the employment agreement with their staff.

Again, doctors themselves differ in their approach to patients and can show distinct bias in their attitudes to certain illnesses, and a moral revulsion can often show through in a medical report. I well remember a colleague of mine showing me a letter which started: 'I am sorry to refer this idiot, he has lazyitis and should have been strangled at birth!' The rest of the letter was very informative and useful, and I am sure the initial sentence was a light-hearted remark designed to warn of trouble ahead, but it could have been taken differently.

It appears to me that in the taking of a medical history such notes as are recorded must take into consideration:

1 permission from the patient;
2 the usefulness of such recordings
   (a) to the recorder,
   (b) to later physicians who may be called on to treat the patient;
3 the possibility of personal bias;
4 the possibility of breaches in confidentiality.

These considerations apply to every medical note ever made, but even more so in the personal field of psychiatry. Almost everyone finds it difficult to relate thoughts of a shocking nature, or embarrassing events in their lives, and yet these, if present, are essential to any analysis. Only when the patient has complete faith in the confidentiality of his revelations will they be forthcoming; seeing the therapist taking notes not only inhibits the verbal confessions but interrupts the patient's flow of conversation.

The use of cameral analysis, however, poses yet another problem where records are concerned.

In Mode One, the verbal analysis of the left hemisphere is accompanied by the acute observation of any pertinent body-language taking place at the same time. This is a very important part of the procedure as it often pinpoints areas of conflict. *Taking notes interrupts the concentration of the therapist and body-language may be missed.*

The method I have followed for years in order to overcome this problem is to tape-record conversation during the session. This serves as an excellent memory bank as well as a source for any written record I may care to make. However, science has added a new dimension, and I now believe that video-recordings are the ideal method to use in Mode One analyses.

With the advent of small, unobtrusive and relatively cheap camcorders, the cassettes of which can be used over and over again, a totally uninterrupted interview is now possible and a written précis can be dictated later at leisure. Editing is simple and quick, and a short, edited version of salient points in interviews could become a valuable part of the patient's notes as well as a unique form of reference.

Apart from the therapist, the video is the only method that can accurately record both human languages, verbal and body, in synchronous apposition and thus detect the presence of possible conflicts between them. A re-run of the video may reveal body-language that had been missed.

With permission from the patient such videos can, and have, provided a teaching source for the recognition of body-language.

Where patients' records are concerned this new dimension should certainly be considered by analysts. Nevertheless, I would not wish to over-emphasize this subject. Cameral analysis is just as effective without any mechanical aids. A small proportion of my cases have been seen through from beginning to end relying entirely on my own memory as source material for letters, notes and so on. The final decision on the choice of method must, of course, be personal to the therapist.

APPROACH TO THE PATIENT

My first words to every patient are to reassure them that whatever they reveal in the course of treatment remains totally between the two of us, and that any information imparted to anyone would be with their permission and would be of a very general nature associated with diagnosis, prognosis and progress in treatment. I indicate the recording apparatus but emphasize that it is used in the place of old-fashioned note-taking and will not be used for any other purpose without permission. When it has served its purpose the tape is wiped clear and used again.

At some convenient point in the first interview I explain to the patient, very briefly, my method of treatment and how I divide it into two modes. I also explain that in Mode One the last quarter of an hour is spent with the patient in hypnosis. During this period no treatment is entered into whatsoever but the sense of total relaxation and the calming effect induced by the method is in itself therapeutic. This period also serves to acquaint the patient with the feeling of this relaxed state and allays any doubt, fear or prejudice they may have harboured. In so doing the patient learns how to go quickly into hypnosis and reach a good working depth necessary for Mode Two.

Occasionally, the more enquiring patient wishes to know more about the state of hypnosis and asks for some form of explanation. 'What is it?', 'Why should it exist?', 'What purpose does it serve?' are typical questions, and to them I find the following neurological explanation helpful.

We have two legs designed to move us about in search of food or to run away from danger. The fact that, because of them, we can play the highly skilled game of football, is merely *a functional spin-off*, they were never developed with football in mind.

We have, throughout our nervous system, two vast neuronal pathways.[9] One is excitatory, the other inhibitory; together they constantly monitor our conscious awareness. For instance, while you are listening to me you are unaware of what is happening to, say, your left foot. Nevertheless, proprioceptive signals are being relayed from this organ giving information on temperature, position-sense, comfort and so on. If all these signals were to arrive at the cortex, the brain would be overwhelmed and concentration impossible. Possession by the central nervous system of an inhibitory mechanism means that only essentially required signals are allowed through to the conscious cortex at any given time. So powerful is this inhibition that even the pain and disability from the fractured collar-bone of the heavily tackled rugby player is ignored in favour of his getting up and hurling himself over the line to score a try. Not until some time later, with release of the inhibitory control, does he realize he has quite a severe injury.

The possibility of inducing altered states of consciousness, such as hypnosis, is, in my opinion, like the ability to play football, *a spin-off* from the possession of an inhibitory mechanism by the central nervous system.

The techniques of Mode One

Mode One is any discussion the therapist has with the patient about the patient's problem, when the patient is in his or her normal, conscious, waking state.

Obviously, it is the first mode of contact the therapist has with the patient, and initially is simply a full medical history followed by a more detailed psychiatric history, *but both must be taken with the patient in full view in order for the therapist to observe the patient's body-language.*

Initially then, the object of Mode One verbal analysis is for the therapist to gain a good impression of the left hemisphere's idea and interpretation of the patient's problem and at the same time to pinpoint potential areas of interhemispheric conflict (discrepancies) for further exploration. In this respect, not only is particular notice taken of the intervention of the right hemisphere through its use of body-language, but also of the patient's dream-language.

Mode One requires the patient to discuss their dreams, past, present or on-going, from which the therapist may glean further information on:

1 the nature of the problem;
2 the symbolic language the patient uses;
3 the progress of the analysis.

Later, when the therapist feels that verbal analysis is as complete as possible and all is ready for Mode Two analysis under hypnosis, Mode One itself takes on a less analytical and more therapeutic role. Nevertheless, during the course of this verbal analysis, *active treatment* of the patient may occur; if it does, it is largely fortuitous and often the result of the triggering of an emotional memory which produces a beneficial effect by the very virtue of its exposure. There is only one rule in cameral analysis, and that is to get the patient better! If an opportunity arises it is up to the therapist to take every advantage of it at whatever point in the analysis it occurs. Unfortunately, these therapeutic gifts are rare; hard work is the norm.

On the other hand, *passive treatment* is going on all the time in this verbal mode. The very fact that 'something is being done' is reassuring. History taking itself has often a 'confessional' quality which may relieve guilt and lessen anxiety. It is also a time in which the patient learns to relax, not only in relation to the therapist, but also within themselves by virtue of the final fifteen minutes of every session being devoted to simple relaxation in the hypnotic state. The patient often volunteers the fact that they feel much better and the problem less of a nuisance, although there is still little, if any, insight.

At this point, Mode One analysis has enabled the therapist to draw up a list of incidents in the life of the patient which are considered of significance to the patient's problem and which require a more detailed emotional investigation. As previously stated, the other method helping in this investigation is the interpretation of the patient's dreams.

This important source of information is gathered mainly by verbal description of dreams past, present and on-going while the patient is in Mode One normal waking state, and a Mode One interpretation of both the manifest and latent content is attempted. However, the latent content may remain a mystery until the whole dream is re-examined under hypnosis. Dream interpretation in cameral analysis is now discussed.

DREAMS AND DREAM INTERPRETATION IN CAMERAL ANALYSIS

From antiquity, individuals of all nations, from philosophers, theologians and scientists to the humblest of citizens, have all voiced their opinions on the origin and function of dreams. Despite this continuous interest, dreams still remain largely a mystery.

Probably the greatest single contribution to dream significance came at the end of the last century with Freud's theory on the interpretation of dreams. Freud considered the dream to be a 'momentous psychic act' concerned with problem solving, and that every dream was 'a disguised fulfilment of a suppressed wish'. He also held that the sexual factor is *always* present in dreams. These have been seen by many as contentious statements, and psychological literature is full of arguments on the pros and cons of such ideas. The great majority, however, have seen his theory of the interpretation of dreams as a brilliant piece of original reasoning and it has remained a milestone in psychological thought since its inception.

One aspect of interpretation which has been universally accepted is his division of the dream into a manifest and a latent content.

The manifest content

This is the obvious and remembered content of the dream. For instance, if the dream was of a pleasant visit to relatives, then this was its manifest content and could be considered as the sole purpose of the dream by anyone to whom it had been related. However, Freud considered that there was another, underlying (latent) meaning.

The latent content

The hidden meaning was often totally different from the obvious meaning. A 'pleasant visit to relatives' could represent the emotional feeling of 'love and recognition'. Such being the case, the dream could be interpreted as a desire for love and recognition.

To the analyst this would suggest that love and recognition were missing from the dreamer's life. If this were so, then this lack might play a significant role in initiating neurotic behaviour, and the correct interpretation of the dream would provide a helpful clue to the understanding of the neurosis.

Cameral analysis utilizes this concept but interprets the manifest and latent contents in terms of left and right hemispheres. It takes the manifest content to be a memory of an actual happening or a phantasy of a happening occurring in the past, and the emotional shroud of this memory to be the latent content. The whole dream is a problem-solving event between the two hemispheres where the latent content is the *pictorial* representation for past situations which contained the emotion needing to be expressed. For example, just as the left hemisphere learns a *WORD* for an *OBJECT* such as a book and can later express this through a verbal or written medium, relying on a memory store for retrieval, so the right hemisphere learns a *SYMBOL* such as the 'bared teeth of a dog' for an *EMOTION* (fear) and can express this emotion in a dream by dreaming of a dog.

Again, a memory store is raided for this expression.

The time when the first experiences of emotions are being laid down in the memory store is in childhood. These, being the first, are of maximum influence, all others being modified by the already learned experience of the first. It is of no wonder to me that childhood memories play such an important part in our lives. They constitute the first learned processes upon which we base the rest of our lives. They should fit in with, or complement, instinctual behaviour such that expected and actual events are as near to each other as possible.

If these memories are too traumatic or do not sufficiently correspond to expected events, then they are shrouded by an anxiety until further learning experience corrects them. If no such learning experience is forthcoming, a chronic anxiety state builds up which may later surface as a behavioural problem or a psychoneurosis. When this happens, of course, the failure of normal learning processes means that the much more difficult process of going back to the original fault and re-learning from that point has to be undertaken. A method incorporating re-educative symptom exposure such as cameral analysis can, by design, effect this purpose.

Freud's concept must be considered a paramount contribution to the understanding of dream psychology, but with the advent of neuropsychology in the last two decades of this century new light has been thrown on the origin, nature and function of both sleep and dreaming.

In 1953, Aserinsky and Kleitman[10] described two stages in sleep distinguished by eye movement: one showed rapid eye movements (REM); the other did not (non-REM). Later, Dement and Kleitman (1957)[11] linked REM sleep with the process of dreaming and showed the latter to be confined to this stage.

Hernandez-Peon (1967)[12] suggested that the neurological basis of dream formation lay in limbic and paleocortical activity. Limbic activity being the origin of the emotional and motivational processes recognized in the dream's *latent content* and neocortical activity causes both relevant remote, and recent, memory processes giving rise to the *manifest content* of dreams. He further suggested that a daily release of the emotional and motivational processes of the limbic system during sleep may prevent them interfering with normal behaviour during the waking state.

David Cohen, in his book *Sleep and Dreaming* (1979),[13] draws attention to a mass of experimental data which suggest that REM dreaming is a function of the right hemisphere. He quotes an unpublished paper by Paul Bakan which draws together far-ranging material from neurological, psychological and psychiatric literature that implicates right hemisphere mediation of dream experience.

He goes on to speculate that the *need* to dream may be directly correlated with the degree of suppression of the right hemisphere during the waking state, when left hemisphere function is dominant and represses that of the right hemisphere. Cohen feels that:

> The question of changes in lateral (Hemispheric) Specialisation during sleep is potentially one of the most exciting, yet one of the least explored issues in sleep research.

From all the above, I believe it could be well argued that dreams are a re-processing phenomena where primitive emotional and motivational processes emanating from the paleomammalian brain are re-structured so as not to clash with logical processes determining waking behaviour. The right hemisphere acts as a 'cortical mediator' between the primitive responses of the limbic system and the logical responses of the left hemisphere. The re-structuring process takes place when the left hemisphere is non-dominant – that is, during sleep – and involves a metaphorical re-run, recognized as dreaming.

If the process is successful, a balanced individual awakes in the morning. If it is only partially successful, a degree of anxiety remains in the individual's waking state, which, depending on its severity, is reflected in psychosomatic symptoms.

Professor Crisp – Crisp et al. (1985);[14] Crisp et al. (1989)[15] – in researching the cause of migraine, puts forward the hypothesis that migraine is the experience of a protective vascular mechanism arising in response to a unilateral cerebral information overload. He feels that, as migraine is a somatic complaint invariably starting just as the patient awakes in the morning, the processes taking place during sleep and designed to even out any hemispheric overload have failed. The resulting unilateral hemispheric overload remains and demands blood-flow to sustain it. This is not acceptable, and a protective vascular reduction in the form of an arterial spasm ensues. Its presence is revealed by the classical unilateral headache with or without visual field disturbances.

One of the interesting aspects of this hypothesis is that it acknowledges the role of sleep as a mediator in information processing. It would also to some extent support the idea that the right hemisphere has the ability to influence the autonomic nervous system when drawing attention to an interhemispheric discrepancy by the use of body-language. The vascular phenomenon of blushing has been previously quoted as an example of such a right hemisphere role.

Cameral analysis theory regards dreams as a metaphorical mani-festation of a re-educative process taking place between logical and emotional ideas of behaviour, the object of the dream process being a resolution of any discrepancies between these ideas which would otherwise prevent their symbiosis.

The interpretation of a dream can point to any unresolved discrepancies and can be a valuable source of information.

Part of this information, like body-language, is from the right hemisphere but is exposed verbally during Mode One analysis. Like body-language, it needs a correct interpretation to be of value. The verbal description of a dream given by the patient contains a manifest content often fairly obvious, but the latent content may still remain much of a mystery. More right hemi-sphere information may be necessary, and it is frequently not until the dream content is re-examined under hypnosis that the latent content becomes apparent.

To illustrate this, a patient of mine, who was a medical graduate working as a hospital registrar and specialising in pathology, came to see me with a problem concerning exams. He had completed all the necessary hospital appointments and was eligible to take the higher fellowship exam which would then entitle him to apply for a consultant post. In fact, he had already taken this exam twice, and on both occasions had failed the viva voce. Evidently he had no problem with the written papers, but when it came to the oral exam he panicked in front of the examiners and failed to answer their questions adequately. There were times when he 'dried up' completely.

This patient suffered with a recurrent nightmare which he felt must be related to his problem; this subsequently proved correct. My patient had passed his first student preliminary exam for his medical degree with extremely good marks, but soon afterwards had his first nightmare in which he dreamed he had failed this exam. In the dream he saw himself dejectedly walking away from the notice-board on which the results were posted. This nightmare recurred on several occasions throughout the rest of his under-graduate days; each time he awoke in a panic. However, he had no trouble in passing further student preliminaries, but when it came to his final exams he felt nervous in the vivas. Nevertheless, he passed his finals with distinction and gained an award in pathology.

About a year after qualifying, the nightmare returned, but this time he dreamed he had failed his finals and saw himself being handed an envelope by an official from the university. The envelope contained details of his exam results showing the subject in which he had failed. In the nightmare he was never able to read the name of the failed subject, it was too blurred.

To me the manifest content of this dream was fairly obvious. It was a classic anxiety dream associated with exams, which is a very common occurrence among all varieties of students the world over. Furthermore, as many old qualified doctors will testify, dreams of failing their finals often recur throughout their lives.

It is as if they have never come to terms with the tensions and anxieties of their clinical years when they meet for the first time tragedy, sadness, disease and death, as well as having to cope with the demands of the examiners. I have read of similar nightmares occurring into very old age in people who had suffered in concentration camps. In their cases it is easy to understand how the extremes of fear and suffering permanently overwhelmed their emotional coping system, and it is a great tribute to the human mind that the mechanisms of maintaining mental stability are as versatile as they are.

My patient's nightmares started, as it were, post-prandially, and were never associated with an actual failure until some eight years later when he came to take his specialist exams. Again he had no problem with his written work; his source of anxiety was a confrontational test, which pointed more to a latent content for an explanation, rather than the manifest content, which was so obviously associated with exams.

The latent content was exposed under hypnosis, when he was asked to imagine himself discussing his nightmare with me. He would feel perfectly relaxed during this discussion, not anxious in any way but merely relating the contents of the nightmare, knowing it to have been a dream and definitely not a reality. At the same time he was told that the content of the dream would be much clearer; for instance, he would be able to identify the subject in which he was purported to have failed. The subject turned out to be obstetrics and gynaecology, but the most revealing factor was that the 'university official' who had handed him the envelope he now clearly recognized as his father. This revelation showed up a latent content in keeping with the emerging analytical picture and enabled the therapeutic course to get quickly under way.

A brief explanation. My patient was afraid of his father, who was a very strict disciplinarian. Throughout my patient's under-graduate days his father had constantly warned him to avoid becoming emotionally involved with any females until he had actually qualified. He feared their distraction could be a negative influence on his son's career and was constantly quoting instances personally known to him where this had occurred. My patient found this an impossible task but was able to keep his secret from his father.

Soon after my patient qualified his father died. Within months my patient introduced to his family, and then married, the girl with whom he had been associating.

Under treatment my patient came to realize, and then accept, that his problem was one of guilt in disobeying his father, which was later aggravated by the addition of feelings of guilt over his father's death.

When he faced his real-life examiners his emotional hemisphere saw them as representing a questioning father, and the questions were on a subject entirely related to females. He could not answer these questions without revealing his guilt, so he dried up.

My patient had no problem in his third attempt at the exam and is now a consultant pathologist.

My object in quoting this case was to show the value of hypnosis in exposing the latent content of dreams and their eventual interpretation to the benefit of treatment strategy. I should add that the brief explanation I have offered was not the complete picture in this case, which included problems in childhood relationships and even choice of career direction.

Chapter 5

Abreaction

One of the major therapeutic aims of cameral analysis is the production of abreactions. What precisely is meant by *abreaction*?

In 1882 Joseph Breuer[1] discovered that, by encouraging patients to re-tell their problems under deep hypnosis, a profound relief of their symptoms often resulted. He called this method *cathartic* and described its therapeutic aim as 'the re-direction of accumulated *affect*, which had become stuck on wrong lines, on to a normal path along which it could obtain discharge (or *abreaction*)' (quoted from *An Autobiographical Study* by S. Freud).

Freud[2] described the practical results of this cathartic procedure as excellent, but stressed the essential nature of a vivid emotional experience in order to obtain a maximum therapeutic response. Later in his life he was to praise the value of abreaction in the hands of Simmel, who used it in the treatment of war neuroses in the German Army during the 1914–18 war. Nevertheless, Freud discarded Breuer's method in favour of the therapeutic method he was developing; he considered the *sexual origin* of a neurosis to be the paramount emotion, and his method – free association and psychoanalysis – to be the treatment of choice. Furthermore, Freud considered that the mysterious element at work behind hypnotism was the *transference situation*, and in order to exclude it, or at least isolate it, it was necessary to *abandon hypnotism*.

This was about 1895, and the fear Freud had of the *hypnotic transference situation* was, in my opinion, both unfounded and unnecessary. It was nevertheless a problem that needed tackling. Freud preferred not to grasp this nettle at this point in his career, although, later, transference became an essential factor in the treatment of patients by psychoanalysis.

It is now well recognized that Freud's abandonment of hypnosis in favour of free association was one of the major factors in causing hypnotherapy (including Breuer's abreactive therapy) to be ignored by the medical profession for nearly a century.

The acute traumatic war neuroses (shell-shock) suffered by soldiers of both armies during the First World War temporarily reinstated the value of *abreactive therapy under hypnosis* as a treatment process. In doing so, it threw fresh light on its mechanism. Whereas previously its success had been ascribed to the revival of repressed, unpleasant memories, it now became obvious that the mere recollection of these incidents was not enough. As originally discovered by Breuer and Freud, the memories had to be accompanied by a profound emotional discharge of associated affect. William Brown (1938),[3] of whom more later, went out of his way to point out that, under hypnosis, *suggestion* may remove the symptom but *abreaction* was essential to remove the cause in order to produce a fully adequate re-association of the mind. One of the most interesting observations was that of Millais Culpin (1920).[4] Culpin, like Brown, had a vast experience of the 1914–18 traumatic war neuroses, and had found that in many cases the causative incident could be easily remembered but its emotional content appeared to have been separated from it and repressed. Continual verbal re-enactment of the memory had simply no effect whatsoever in these cases, but, under hypnosis, it was possible to uncover and abreact the repressed emotional trauma with a resulting immediate improvement in the patient's condition. If we consider this finding of Culpin in terms of cameral analysis, the verbal, non-emotional memory of the left hemisphere remained available for verbal recall at all times, but the right hemisphere's emotional memory of the same incident was too horrific to sustain and might have contained memories of the imminent approach of certain death. Under hypnosis, the right hemisphere's emotional memory is revealed and abreacted in what have now become survival conditions; the subject's intense fear of death, frozen in time by the action of repression, is released in the knowledge of his survival; dissociation becomes integration, and the two hemispheres function normally again.

I deliberately mention the concept of certain death or mutilation in this context because, where acute traumatic war neuroses are concerned, the majority of cases contained this element. In peacetime, however (except for rare natural disasters such as earthquakes), such extremes of fear as experienced by soldiers subjected to many hours of continuous shellfire would be an impossible occurrence. The 1914–18 war exposed human behaviour under these conditions to psychological and psychiatric analysis on an unprecedented scale, and, in my opinion, gave a profound insight into the mechanics of brain-function with particular reference to the origins of its defence mechanisms. Sadly, with only a few notable exceptions, this knowledge was neglected by the medical profession; it was given another chance with the outbreak of the Second World War in 1939.

Between the wars one of these notable exceptions was Dr William Brown, Director of the Institute of Experimental Psychology at the University of Oxford. Brown had been the neurologist to the Fourth Army British Expeditionary Force in France in the First World War and subsequently the Medical Officer in charge of Craiglockhart War Hospital for Neurasthenic Officers. He had vast experience of both front-line and long-term treatment of the war neuroses, or what we would now call Post-Traumatic Stress Disorder (PTSD). He considered shell-shock to be a dissociated state produced by a profound mental shock, which in turn caused symptoms of physical dissociation. More interestingly, he found that hypnosis *quickly* cured these cases *if they were treated soon after the onset of symptoms*. The longer they were left in their dissociated state, the more difficult it was to re-associate them.

Brown's method was to encourage the soldier to re-live his experiences under hypnosis with great emotional vividness. The result was that the dissociation disappeared and the patient became quickly and completely re-associated, so much so that some 70 per cent of such cases were soon able to rejoin their unit.

He describes a typical early case referred to him within hours of the onset of the symptoms, and comments '*such cases I saw by the hundred near the firing-line during the European War*'.[5]

Here is Brown's vivid description of shell-shock:

> The patient would be brought into hospital lying on a stretcher, perhaps dumb, trembling violently, perspiring profusely, his face showing an expression of great terror, his eyes either with a fixed stare or rolling from side to side. When one questioned him and got him to answer in writing, he would tell one that he was quite unable to remember what happened to him. In some way or another he had been knocked out, and had come-to to

find that he was paralysed and could not speak. That is a case of acquired hysteria – hysteria produced by a mental shock caused by a shell explosion. Why do we say that it is hysteria? Because we have come to restrict the term 'hysteria' to a form of mental illness characterized by crude functional dissociation.

The man I have described was in a dissociated state. If one considers the personality as a system of psycho-physical powers, such as the power of walking, the power of talking, the powers of hearing and seeing, the power of controlling expression of the emotions, the power of remembering the events of the past, and other powers, one will find that in the hysteric one or more of the powers has become split off or dissociated from the total personality.

In the case I have just described in general terms there is such a functional dissociation. The patient has lost the powers of recalling a certain set of memories, viz. those corresponding to the experience of the shell explosion and of what followed immediately thereupon.

He has also lost the power of speaking and the power of walking; he has lost the power of controlling the manifestations of fear – he cannot control his tremors; his nervous system has also lost the power of controlling another manifestation of fear, viz. profuse perspiration; and on investigation one may find other losses of power, e.g. he may have lost sensitivity in the lower limbs, his lower limbs may be numb. In such a case as that we may believe that it was the mental shock that produced the dissociation.

Moreover, the dissociation was not only a mental dissociation it was also a physical dissociation. Certain parts of the cerebral cortex had become functionally disconnected from other parts, so that the cerebral cortex, the part of the brain we may take as directly related to conscious experience, did not work in its entirety. Certain parts were working independently of other parts, or were not working while other parts were working. It was thus a physical dissociation as well as a mental one. If we try to imagine what sort of a dissociation this is on the physical side, we feel irresistibly compelled to think of it as a breaking across of nerve-conducting paths. We know that, in general, the nervous system is made up of cells and fibres (neurons) joining one another at the synapses. These nerve fibres are not in contact with one another, but there is a minute gap between one nerve fibre and the next. This is called a synapse.

When the nervous system functions normally, the impulse can jump across that gap.

Under special conditions, such as fatigue, the influence of drugs, etc., some of these gaps may be so increased in resistance that the impulse cannot pass. In the case of acquired hysteria, where there is a functional dissociation, we may assume that some of these synapses have begun to offer more resistance than usual. The nerve fibres may have contracted, so that the gap has become greater than before, or some other change may have taken place in the nervous tissue.

That would be the explanation on the physical side. We can say that it is (in general) the explanation, inasmuch as it fits in with what we know otherwise of the functioning of the nervous system. I have described it in some detail because I wanted to illustrate my previous statement that when there is a functional disturbance of the nervous system there is also a structural change. Even in such a functional disturbance as acquired hysteria there is a structural change. Mental dissociation corresponds to physical dissociation.

Now we find that cases of this kind are easy to hypnotize, and that they are most quickly cured by (even) light hypnosis.

This description and his explanation of the mechanics of PTSD showed Dr William Brown to be not only a shrewd observer, but a far-thinking neurologist who was already anticipating the results of future research into the neurophysiological and neuropsychological workings of the brain. Furthermore, his vast experience in the use of hypnosis led him to have no doubt whatsoever of the great therapeutic value of abreaction.

He deplored those in psychoanalytic circles who belittled its value and who tried to explain its beneficial effect in terms of transference. He illustrated his opposition to this Freudian concept by quoting a case[6] where the patient himself induced a beneficial abreaction without recourse to any therapist. Transference could in no way have played a part in such a situation!

Another psychiatrist, working between the wars, was J.S. Horsley. In 1936 Horsley[7] developed a technique which he described as 'short-cut psychotherapy', in which patients, under the influence of intravenous pentothal (a barbiturate anaesthetic drug injected into the veins), were encouraged to re-live traumatic events that had occurred in their lives. Horsley gave this drug-induced abreactive technique the name of *narco-analysis* (literally, drug-analysis) and, to me, the method is interesting in that it closely parallels cameral analysis in certain aspects. Both are analytical and encourage the abreaction of past events, events which may have contributed to the abnormal psychological state of the patient. Both are used in the treatment of the psychoneuroses in general as opposed to the confines of PTSD. Both narco-analysis and hypnosis probably owe their results to their action in some way on the septo-hippocampal system of the brain.[8] The barbiturates succeed more by direct action at a synaptic level, and hypnosis through the inhibitive action of the reticular activating system stimulated from the frontal cortex.[9] Both are known to affect the frequency of theta rhythm, which can be used as a measure of septo-hippocampal function; inhibition of this function seems to lead to a reduction of anxiety.[10]

Unfortunately, narco-analysis had little or no impact in the world of psychotherapy until it was picked up by psychiatrists such as Sargant and Slater[11] in 1940 and used by them in the treatment of shell-shock (PTSD) in Dunkirk survivors. Later, as the war progressed, the inhaled anaesthetic, ether, was substituted for pentothal.

As I mentioned in the Introduction to this book, I was fortunate, as a medical student in 1946, to witness the treatment of some of these acute war neuroses by abreactive techniques. Among the psychiatrists involved in these procedures were a few who considered that abreactions produced under hypnosis were safer and more reliable. The drawback of intravenous pentothal lay in its administration; the speed at which it was given and the amount injected were critical and the margin of error was small. When it was given too slowly, the patient often appeared drunk and confused, making communication difficult; if it was given too quickly, the patient seemed almost anaesthetized and no abreaction ensued.

The anaesthetic vapour, ether, on the other hand, produced such a degree of excitatory reaction that the patient had to be physically restrained, either by attendants or a strait-jacket, to avoid any injury occurring.[12] Nevertheless, abreactions obtained under ether were often spectacular and ended up with a total emotional collapse. Whenever this occurred, recovery was often rapid and more complete. Sargant and Shorvon (1945)[13] likened this emotional collapse to the transmarginal inhibition exhibited by Pavlov's dogs after the trauma they experienced in the Leningrad floods. They suggested that an explanation of the recovery of patients by abreaction could be made in terms of Pavlovian theory.

At the risk of a slight diversion, I think it fitting to take a brief glance at Pavlov's extraordinary work. Using research methods that could never have been tolerated in this country, Pavlov was able to show that it was possible to induce behavioural patterns in dogs. Furthermore, once these patterns (conditioned reflexes) were established, experiments designed to break them down produced severe anxiety states in these animals. Moreover, by producing a complete mental confusion, total *reversal* of previous behavioural patterns could be observed. The significance of these findings, if they could be related to human behaviour, was not lost on the post-revolutionary Soviet Union.

The political hierarchy made use of them in the ideological struggle then occurring both inside and outside their country. So it came about, through Pavlov's work, that the Soviets developed and perfected the 'brain-washing' technique seen to be so effective in the state trials of the 1930s. An amazed world witnessed the sight of intelligent and renowned figures genuinely confessing to criminal acts against the state, or voicing ideological dogma in a total reversal of their previously held values.

The enormous importance of the Pavlovian theory was not confined to political indoctrination but could also be applied to the explanation of other sudden psychological 'conversions', such as the adoption of a religious belief following an emotional catharsis, the ecstasy of divine revelations, certain 'possession' states, and, as Shorvon and Sargant suggested, to the *therapeutic value of abreaction*.

When Pavlov subjected his dogs to what he termed 'transmarginal stimulation' (stresses and conflicts beyond their endurance limits), he produced a condition he termed '*transmarginal inhibition*', and the characteristics of this mental breakdown were very similar to that of shell-shock in humans. In this state paradoxical behaviour was apparent; for example, food previously shunned was eaten and food previously preferred was ignored. In humans, if left in this state, similar paradoxical behaviour could be elicited both physically and mentally and, indeed, could be encouraged by suggestion. The possibility of 'brain-washing' was there for all to see!

This high suggestibility also accounted for the ease with which humans, in this extreme state of cortical inhibition (that is, shell-shock), could be hypnotized, and Shorvon and Sargant were quick to point out that by inducing an excitatory response under hypnosis this inhibition could be overcome.

They therefore postulated that abreaction of the intense events leading up to shell-shock *could rupture the recently acquired pattern of conditioned behaviour* and *may have some relation to the therapeutic value of emotional abreaction in psychotherapeutic techniques*. I have no reason to contradict this theory but would like to comment on it in terms of cameral analysis.

Pavlov considered conditioned reflexes to be part of the learning process and as such to involve the brain *cortices*. (The non-conditioned reflexes are *sub-cortical*, originating in the lower centres of the limbic system and brain-stem; they are instinctual and involve fundamental behaviour associated with survival, defence of territory and mating. They are genetically transmitted and can be modified by *cortical* control.)

As I have previously mentioned, it is my opinion that shell-shock (acute war neuroses and PTSD are both names for the same mental state) is a dissociative phenomenon resulting from intense inhibitory activity of the *cortex*. Emotional thoughts of extreme intensity, involving certain mutilation and death, have to be 'blocked out' in order for the individual mentally to survive at the time the stress is occurring. The enormity of the inhibiting process represses both motor and sensory function, such as speech, limb control, skin sensation, memory and so on, producing an almost total lack of brain co-ordination. (This emergency measure is brought about by activation of inhibitory processes such as the reticular formation, and this may also account for the ease with which hypnosis can be induced in these individuals.) It is possible that, in the course of abreacting the event, a re-education of the memory takes place; the individual realizes he has survived, repression (inhibition) is no longer necessary and a re-association of the cortex ensues.

If the shell-shock remains *untreated*, the symptoms gradually become an integral part of the individual's learned behaviour, rather similar to a conditioned reflex; the result is that they

become more permanently patterned and thus more difficult to
eradicate.

Up to this point, in answering the question 'What precisely is
meant by abreaction?', I have confined my definition to 'the recall
of past events in a person's life and the revival and *expression* of
the emotional content of that experience'. So far, I have illustrated
this by historical reference to the treatment of the acute war
neuroses arising in the twentieth century. I have done this deliberately because shell-shock is a 'pure' condition arising in apparently
well-orientated individuals and the result of a known, extreme,
psychological trauma. There is no doubt as to how, why and when
it occurred; nor is there any argument as to the main presenting
symptoms, which are always of an acute, dissociative type and the
result of massive inhibitory stimulation of the cortex. I totally
accept that this extreme mental condition is rarely seen outside
war situations or horrific peacetime disasters, but the importance
lies in its response to treatment. I hope I have been able to show
that abreacting these events is highly effective, and that quick and
permanent resolution of the symptoms has been very well
documented.

*Can abreactive treatment be equally effective in other nervous
conditions where there has been* no *obvious, massive, initiating
trauma?*

I believe it can. Furthermore, I believe that abreaction is a
normal, natural, integrative mechanism, part of the learning process, and can be seen at work in the function of dreams. It forms
an important part of treatment based on cameral analysis.

Again, in my opinion, mental dissociation itself is an emergency
protective device and is associated with the mechanism of repression; both of these, in turn, are themselves an integral part of
memory and learning processes. It is rather like a power cut; when
the system as a whole is overloaded, parts are shut off in order of
their priority.

A child, coming into contact with a sudden alarming situation of
which it has not had any previous experience, automatically sets
in motion learning processes. For instance, a six-year-old child
calls at the home of a new school-friend for the first time. He
knocks on the door. It is opened by the mother of his new friend.
As she opens the door a large Alsatian dog bounds out from
behind her straight towards the child. The dog is nearly as big
as the child and certainly as heavy. Taken off balance the child is

knocked over by the dog and is clearly very frightened. The mother grabs the dog, scolds it, and pushes it back into the house and turns to pick up and comfort the child. She reassures him that the dog is quite harmless, that the dog only wished to play, and that he must come in to meet the family, which includes the dog. With this assurance, and being in the arms of an adult, fear quickly abates; by the end of the morning the incident is apparently forgotten and both children and the dog are playing happily together.

Over lunch in his own home the child relates his morning activities to his mother. He says that his friend has a big dog that is very friendly and allows them to ride on its back, that they played with his friend's trains but the dog had to be put in another room because it kept chasing the trains. When they had their elevenses his friend put a sugar-lump on the dog's nose and the dog just sat with it on his nose until his friend said 'eat it', whereupon the dog tossed the lump in the air and caught it. 'It must be a clever dog,' said the mother, pleased that her son had very obviously enjoyed the morning.

The child had made no mention of the incident at the door.   .

Why no mention?

Learning processes had been at play that morning, and by the time the child left for his lunch he had enjoyed himself and would have liked to go again. His logical fear of the dog had completely abated, so it could be argued that there was no need for him to tell his mother. On the other hand, the child could have reasoned that, were his mother to know, she might have been less inclined to allow him to go to that house again; but this would have been left hemisphere logic and therefore more likely to be conscious. In fact, the child had no conscious knowledge of why he did not mention the incident. One can assume that learning processes had reconciled the fear by subsequent events and logically he was happy with the experience. However, emotionally there was still some way to go. The *memory* of the initial shock was there but the verbal hemisphere repressed it when describing the morning's events. The child's emotional hemisphere did its utmost to reveal this by constantly forcing the *subject of the dog* into his conversation over lunch with his mother, but the verbal hemisphere kept strict control by verbally removing all threat from the dog. This, after all, was logically correct in so far as that particular dog was shown to be harmless.

In this learning process it is as if the logical left hemisphere had told the emotional right hemisphere that it had been silly to be frightened that morning because it had misinterpreted the dog's exuberance as dangerous instead of playful. Therefore, there was no need to condemn the dog for what was the right hemisphere's own emotional error.

This learning process had worked unconsciously and by the use of repression had prevented a logical misunderstanding arising. There still remained, however, an emotional *memory of fear* associated with the shape of a very large Alsatian dog. It is possible that the reason why the child failed to mention the incident is that the fear involved was sufficient to produce a temporary dissociation of the event in his mind, almost as if he had fainted at the time and had come round a few minutes later with no knowledge of the event.

This would be analogous to the dissociation seen after PTSD but on a very much smaller scale.

Time would reveal this possibility. If, in subsequent years, the child or young adult developed an irrational fear of large Alsatian dogs (as opposed to other large dogs), or felt apprehensive when approaching the front door of any strange house for the first time, then this behaviour would favour such an explanation. If this anxiety was such as to warrant treatment, then explorative regression under hypnosis, with recall and abreaction of the incident, might be necessary to produce a therapeutic re-association.

However, for the moment let us consider that this child's experience was of minimal mental trauma and that subsequent events were sufficient to quell the anxiety quickly, so much so that by lunchtime he had mentally come to terms with it and it was verbally forgotten.

But was it *emotionally forgotten*?

The answer is certainly not! Furthermore, it still remains an *emotional error* in the form of an incorrect interpretation of 'danger' instead of 'playfulness'. This emotional error still has to be altered or diminished to an extent that negates any conflict between the hemispheres. The left hemisphere has to cease to consider the right hemisphere to be 'silly' (that is, illogical), which had necessitated the left hemisphere applying a verbal censorship; the right hemisphere must in turn release its anxiety content, which was the illogical part. How is this done?

In my opinion the child has literally to 'sleep on it'. The day's events are sorted out in sleep. Dreams are the conciliatory mechanism that solve discrepancies between the two hemispheres.

How can I justify this statement? I certainly cannot prove it!

The clue lies in the phenomenon of shell-shock (PTSD) and its undeniable response to treatment by abreaction under hypnosis.

It is my opinion that dreams are a re-run of past events in which the events are relived in symbolic form by the right hemisphere. In this re-run, emotional feelings are abreacted and re-associated to come in line with the more logical thought-processing of the left hemisphere.

To re-state this in other terms.

I believe that dreams are re-educative processes involving hindsight, in which primitive survival reactions are emotionally reframed into a less anxious and more understandable mode, producing a more composed individual.

If this is so, then it would follow that abreaction itself is a natural mechanism involved in mental learning and control. It would also follow that by encouraging the abreaction of past events a therapeutic insight could be the response.

So the child went to bed that night. Later, he became restless in his sleep. Later still, his mother heard him cry out in his sleep and went into his room to comfort him saying: 'Everything is fine, don't worry, it was only a dream.' The child settled and a peaceful night ensued.

The next morning, and prompted by his mother's enquiry, the child related the following dream:

> I was walking to school when some boys started throwing stones at me. I picked up a stone and threw it back at them and the boys went away. Then you came along and said, 'That's fine, you have won!' I think it was a game we were all playing and my stone hit the target. I was very pleased.

In my opinion this dream corrected the emotional error of *danger* by re-structuring the emotional scene from *anxiety* to one of *pleasure*. Both hemispheres were now in agreement, and any possible threat to mental stability in the form of an anxiety neurosis (such as a future dog-phobia) had been diminished or even overcome by natural mechanisms.

One of the mechanisms was the emotional abreaction of the dog incident in the symbolic form of a dream – a dream, which appears totally unrelated to the actual incident when described verbally, but when analysed emotionally is a total re-run. The right hemisphere has no vocabulary and cannot use words to evoke emotion. Instead, it chooses scenes with a similar emotional content, just as in mime where the wiping away of imaginary tears invokes a feeling of sorrow in the audience.

Subjecting this simple dream to cameral analysis, we have the left (verbal) hemisphere's description, which, as previously intimated, conjures up a scene unrelated to any other.

But let us look at the right hemisphere's emotional 'description'.

Going to school   =   emotion of slight apprehension
Throwing stones   =   emotion of fear due to danger
Being comforted   =   emotion of feeling of protection
Winning the game =   pleasure

This analysis is an exact replica of the emotional content of the dog incident except for the end-result, which is one of pleasure and not anxiety.

In the dream, 'going to school' symbolizes the child's visit to his school-friend's house. The fear and danger invoked by the dog is symbolized in the stone-throwing threat. The comfort of the school-friend's mother is represented in the dream by his own mother. *But* . . . the purpose of the dream is to re-structure the emotion and it does this by converting the fear of stone-throwing into a game which the dreamer won and was pleased! – pleasure, not anxiety!

At this point a critic may rightly observe that other interpretations of this dream are possible. It may well be, for instance, that the child *was* anxious about stone-throwing schoolboys and that the comfort obtained *was indeed* that of his real mother when she visited his room. In the dream there is no *obvious* connection with any dog. This is a very legitimate argument and throws into focus the whole question of dream interpretation. I favour my interpretation of the dream because the name of the dog was 'Winston'!

Dreaming, like hypnosis, is an extraordinary phenomenon and its influence has played an immeasurable part in the affairs of humans. It has been a constant part of their philosophy and enquiry throughout recorded time. In the meanwhile, by drawing attention to the abreactive element in dreams I hope I have shown why I consider abreaction to be a normal mental mechanism involved in the learning and re-structuring processes and, *ipso facto*, of therapeutic value.

Stimulating the abreaction of a past event or events under hypnosis is not necessarily a simple matter; there is no infallible set of procedural rules to help the therapist. Whereas in shell-shock the cause is immediate and known and the abreaction of the events relatively easy to stimulate, childhood trauma, occurring twenty or more years previously, has been covered by so many other related anxieties that each one has to be peeled off like the layers of an onion-skin until the core problem emerges. On top of this, even when the therapist is almost 100 per cent positive that a certain trauma is the root of the patient's neurosis, an apparent abreaction of the event inexplicably seems to have simply no therapeutic effect. I believe there is an explanation for this finding and patience at this point is paramount.

Mental protective mechanisms are very cleverly formulated from learned experience, and, once established, can be used repeatedly throughout life in varying circumstances. Unfortunately, wrong reasoning or wrong behaviour – that is, behaviour considered to be outside the norm of the ethnic group of which the individual is a member – can become legitimized in the reasoning of that individual if such behaviour results in a positive secondary gain. In other words, the secondary gain resulting from the initial error becomes itself the prime stimulus for repeating the error. In my opinion, abreaction of this 'legitimized' guilt may have little or no therapeutic effect because there is little or no interhemispheric imbalance to be corrected. To give an example.

A nine-year-old boy, riding pillion on his elder brother's bicycle, entangles his left foot in the rear wheel spokes. The ankle is severely twisted and a deep cut sustained. The injury is painful. He is off school for two weeks. He derives considerable sympathy from his family and friends. His elder brother is blamed for the accident because he did not warn his younger brother to keep his feet away from the wheel, but the injured child knows that, in truth, it was he who was to blame. He was trying to make a rattling sound by putting his shoe on the spokes, rather like running a stick along railings!

The learning processes in this single incident are many. The left hemisphere has a verbal memory for immediate recall but represses any mention of the stick/railing effect.

The emotional memories of the right hemisphere are more

compartmentalized and consist of guilt for not exonerating his brother, but satisfaction in terms of sibling rivalry; an emotional memory of his parents' anxiety; the sympathy from his friends combined with a feeling of exultation in being briefly their centre of conversation, and so on and so forth.

The passage of time and the healing of the wound produce a *physical* rehabilitation. *Emotional* equilibrium is achieved by dream processes over this period, and when he returns to school a fortnight later all appears back to normal, albeit he is a wiser individual.

Two years later, now aged eleven, the child who had the accident is encouraged to join a Scout camp for fourteen days in his summer holidays. To him this sounds a great idea and he really looks forward to the adventure.

It is his first time away from home.

Unfortunately, the organization has slipped up with the accommodation and he is put into a tent with much older boys whom he does not know; they are very off-hand with him. He becomes terribly homesick.

His logical hemisphere tells him to 'stop being a cry-baby' and to 'stick it out', but the emotion of homesickness is too strong and a compromise must be reached. Logically, he is not allowed to be a 'cry-baby' in such a male company and feels guilty, but emotionally he needs the attention of friends, the safety of home surroundings, and some understanding. Learning processes have provided him with a previous painful emotional pattern which could effect such a compromise but this involved an injured ankle.

Later that day he failed to turn up for lunch and the scoutmaster found him upset and in tears in the tent. Between the sobs he related that he had slipped and twisted his left ankle. The scoutmaster could not find any evidence of swelling but noticed the old scars and is told of the previous injury. Under these circumstances, and particularly as the boy is so upset, he wisely packs the boy off home.

Once home the injured ankle miraculously recovers.

The secondary gain of the original injury has been used by the child to solve a new primary emotional problem without exposing its origin.

Another layer, another 'onion-skin', has been added to a core guilt.

Six years later, the child, now a young adolescent under considerable pressure from his parents to achieve good results in his school-leaving certificate, drags his left leg for no apparent reason; but because there had been a recent case of poliomyelitis in the town he was isolated for a month, which prevented him sitting his exams. The leg made a complete recovery soon after the exams. He was later awarded his certificate on the results of his mock exams held earlier in the year. This gave him grades lower than his parents had expected but, as the latter explained to their friends, 'It was really very bad luck for him particularly as he had worked so hard up to the exams and he had a terrible cold when he took his mocks!'

Fourteen years later, as a married man of thirty-one, he came to me as a patient. He was suffering from a partially paralysed left leg. A thorough neurological examination revealed no physical cause for the paralysis and the diagnosis of a conversion hysteria was made. When in the hypnotic state he could walk well without any sign of weakness in either leg.

To continue with this patient's history. He left school to become articled to an accountant. He found his qualifying exams a struggle but he eventually passed them and obtained a job in the City. He married a girl from the typing pool who had been sent to his firm as a temporary employee to cover for staff on holiday. She was unaccustomed to the work and found it difficult; as a result she was frequently criticized. My patient was the only one who helped and encouraged her. Their relationship continued after she returned to the typing pool and they were married some two years later.

One of my patient's problems was that he lacked confidence in himself, which spilt over into his work. This led to his being considered a fairly ineffectual individual, and promotion was slow.

He was frequently overtaken in this matter by younger members of the firm. His wife eventually realized his position and became critical. An undercurrent of dissatisfaction, already present, turned to a brooding bitterness and, without informing his firm, but with the full approval of his wife, he began applying for other posts being offered in the City. Unfortunately, several unsuccessful interviews drained his confidence yet further, he gave up applying and settled down to accept his position, persuading himself that after all he was working for a good firm and being paid a good salary. This decision altered his attitude; he became more amenable and slowly developed a greater liking for his work. For a while his future looked brighter, but sadly this was not to continue.

The blow came when his immediate boss left the firm and a very bright junior was promoted to the vacant post. After a short settling-in period the new boss became more confident of his position, and as his authority grew he became less tolerant of my patient. The situation gradually deteriorated into a mutual dislike and my patient became depressed.

The dislike turned to hatred and bitterness returned. My patient felt in a trap. His previous lack of success in changing his job meant to him that he could see no way out of his present post. He tried to argue with himself that logically he had a wife and responsibilities and needed to work. Emotionally, he hated every minute of his working day and wanted to quit. He solved this hemispheric conflict by partially paralysing his left leg, which satisfied both hemispheres; to the outside world he did not appear to be shirking his responsibilities, nor was he going to work.

The same behavioural pattern had been used to solve an emotional problem, but clearly this time the seriousness of his situation demanded a better solution. His coping mechanism, relying as it did on the error of utilizing a secondary gain from an injury, was an inadequate answer for an adult with mature responsibilities. Followed to its logical conclusion, a partially paralysed leg would so damage the quality of his life that the cure he was attempting by paralysing his leg would be worse than the disruption the cause had initiated.

Therapy depended on the re-educative symptom exposure of his coping mechanisms. From his history I believed that this would involve the abreaction of his dragging leg at the time of his exams, and his sprained ankle at the Scout camp. But although on several occasions he clearly age-regressed well to both these events and appeared to be re-living the scenes, neither abreaction produced any improvement in his leg movement. This was most disappointing because it seemed to me that these events were an obvious source of conflict.

Where was I wrong?

The answer became clear with the abreaction of the bicycle ride and the emotional elements associated with it. There was an immediate improvement, and the patient stated that he felt his leg belonged to him again. Six months later, but admittedly in much changed circumstances which must have contributed to the cure, his left leg moved normally.

To me the explanation of why on occasions there appears to be no response to abreaction of previous events may lie in the concept of secondary gain.

I have come to the conclusion that the re-living of a secondary gain may not necessarily expose the source of the gain. Only exposure of the original incident that led to the initial error in the learning mechanism allows re-structuring to take place and the road to recovery to commence. The initial error was the erroneous idea that a damaged ankle was learnt as an 'advantage' in solving certain emotional problems.

This is not to deny the value of secondary gain. To me it is a normal, natural and valuable learning mechanism, but it has a built-in Achilles heel. Three months after his leg first started to drag it still remained a problem and he continued to be off work. His firm was naturally interested in his prognosis and correctly asked for their own medical opinion. This was granted, and the firm, at their expense, employed an independent neurologist to make a report. Soon after receiving it the firm made my patient redundant but on very generous terms which served to soften the blow.

In the process of re-structuring, my patient had been encouraged to re-examine his life and, in particular, his job.

By the time his redundancy was announced he had already decided to change direction and was considering a less demanding job with the then GPO. Nevertheless, his sacking came as a shock, and when I saw him soon afterwards he was still angry. I think his first words to me on that occasion are worth mentioning, as they illustrate a right hemisphere communication by metaphor.

My patient was a very keen cricket spectator and frequently travelled long distances to watch a match. His knowledge of the cricket scene was immense and he frequently used cricket terms in his conversation. When he made his way into my room with the help of his walking-stick, he dropped into the chair and said: 'I've been bowled leg before wicket!'

His emotional hemisphere had said it all! The words were merely a borrowed brush with which to paint the picture!

I have used this case history to explain the mechanism I believe to be at work when apparently successful abreactions produce disappointing results, but it does serve to illustrate another therapy factor.

Soon after he was sacked, the bicycle incident was unearthed and abreacted. He immediately felt that his leg 'belonged' to him again, which turned out to be the start of his recovery process, but it was a full six months later before he would accept that his leg was no longer a problem.

During this period of re-structuring he discovered many things about himself that he had never suspected and he developed a more accurate identity. For instance, as a child he took pianoforte lessons and really enjoyed them. His teacher was most encouraging and stimulated his enthusiasm saying that he was a very natural player and should do well. Unfortunately, the family moved, and as so often happens in the ensuing upheaval, promising opportunities are lost, or delayed to such an extent that they become lost. This happened to my patient.

When his potential in this field came out in his history I quickly pounced on it and encouraged him to take up the piano again, ostensibly to fill in the time enforced by his relative immobility. He saw some sense in this and found that playing calmed his general level of anxiety; music once more became an important part of life and his enjoyment.

Music is primarily a function of the emotional right hemisphere, and its re-introduction at that stage of his treatment may have played a much greater part in his recovery than one would give credit.

Similarly he realized that he had been virtually forced into accountancy by his school careers master, who appeared to rely entirely on assessment through school subjects. More often than not this is a very accurate method but, because of the Western nations' emphasis on left hemisphere learning, children with right hemisphere potentials are often at a disadvantage. If lucky they emerge eventually as 'late developers'.

It was too late for my patient to start a totally different career, but his change in direction to the then GPO made good use of his training. The relief he experienced when he suddenly realized that the decision he had made to change direction was obviously so right and there was no blame or criticism attached must also have contributed to his recovery.

I cannot close this chapter without mentioning spontaneous abreaction.

This is a condition in which the hypnotized patient, without any prompting from the therapist, abreacts some previous life experience. It occurs suddenly and without warning, and may surprise an unexpecting therapist into terminating the session, particularly if the patient indulges in a lot of physical movement and noise. The more experienced therapist will recognize the condition and make good use of it, giving the patient full encouragement to complete the abreaction until calm ensues. Spontaneous abreaction must be considered as a gift from the patient to the therapist. It often highlights the underlying problem and may cut hours of therapist's time as well as being beneficial to the patient.

It was once a gift to me as a tutor. I was demonstrating age regression to an audience of about eighty medical and dental practitioners at the Whittington Hospital in London when one of the four hypnotized volunteers, relaxing on chairs in front of the rest of the audience, went into a spontaneous abreaction. Considerable emotion was expressed before the abreaction ended in quiet sobbing.

The reaction of the audience was interesting. Some were visibly taken aback, while others were obviously uncomfortable. All were relieved when calm ensued and the session terminated.

Discussion of the incident went on at intervals throughout the week-end and the impact of this quite accidental demonstration was most noticeable. It really underlined the value of hypnosis in uncovering repressed emotion.

I might add that if volunteers in the course of a demonstration exhibit signs of discomfort, the correct procedure is to follow them up in a later session to make sure that no undue anxieties have been aroused.

The particular volunteer I have mentioned turned out to be a very normal and well-orientated individual with no significant problems. The incident abreacted had occurred in childhood and, interestingly, had been the source of an occasional nightmare. The coping mechanism was still at work, but I felt that any extra help or interference was quite unnecessary.

Spontaneous abreaction can occur without hypnosis, but usually the individual is in some form of altered consciousness or has taken drugs such as sodium amytal. I well remember a Hurricane pilot who had been shot down in the Battle of Britain frequently abreacting the event in the most unlikely places, such as at the back of a Cambridge omnibus. Although his physical injuries were of a minor nature the horror of baling out of a burning aircraft caused a mental breakdown which resulted in his being invalided out of the RAF. Some six months later he was sufficiently re-covered to resume his war-interrupted university studies.

I was a fellow student at the time, and the abreactive exploits of this ex-pilot were a source of much conversation and certainly stimulated my lifelong interest in the phenomenon. Now, and with hindsight, I see his abreactions as a continuing process of mental rehabilitation which, by the time he had taken his degree, must have been virtually complete, because during his time in Cambridge the attacks gradually diminished and then disap-peared. As far as I was aware, any formal psychiatric treatment had ceased as soon as he left the RAF – but he did have a very nice girlfriend!

Chapter 6

Cameral analysis and art form

By 'art form' I mean any non-verbal creative work such as two-dimensional drawings, paintings, photography, or three-dimensional sculpture, which includes architecture, fashion design, mechanical invention and so on. Music, of course, is art form in a less tangible state (unless one considers the musical score itself as a tangible representation), and because of this special dimension it is discussed separately.

In cameral analysis art form, like dreams and body-language, is another method by which the right hemisphere finds expression for its thoughts and feelings, and as such can be used as follows:

Analytically

1 As an uncovering agent. Each work of art has, like dreams, a manifest and a latent content, and can be similarly interpreted to expose any interhemispheric discrepancies.
2 In the understanding of the right hemisphere's philosophy or attitude to life. For example, a religious theme can be, or has been, expressed in pagan myths. Or, more simply, attitude can be shown as a plain expression of so-called fact by a patient. For instance, a self-portrait drawn by an anorexic depicts a grossly fat little figure whereas in truth the figure is pathetically thin.

Therapeutically

1 To dispose of guilt by representing a sin as a metaphor in art form and then destroying this image either literally or metaphorically.
2 Similar to an abreaction, by utilizing the catharsis associated with creativity.
3 As a source of metaphysical or divine power in which an art form is endowed with the supernatural force of the being or beings it represents.

To illustrate the analytical use of art, I would like to take a well-known, classical painting by Sandro Botticelli, painted in the fifteenth century and part of the collection of the National Gallery in London. The picture has the title *Venus and Mars* (see Figure 6.1).

To anyone coming across it for the first time and knowing nothing about it other than the title, it is nevertheless a very fine, eye-catching painting. It exhibits a superb expertise in the use of paint in depicting the detail of the hair and dress of Venus and the metallic texture of the armour and helmet of Mars. The composition of the figures and the clever use of the background to throw the foreground into high relief along with the mischievous antics of the wood-nymphs all add to giving it the stamp of a masterpiece.

Because of its title we can say that the manifest content of the picture depicts the occasion in Greek mythology when the god Mars (god of War) seduces the goddess Venus (goddess of Love). Judging by the exhausted and naked state of Mars, the seduction has already taken place. He is so completely fatigued that not even the vigorous blowing of a conch-horn into his right ear stirs him, whereas, in stark contrast, the tranquillity of Venus gives her an almost bored air. This suggests another meaning to the painting which, because it was certainly a meaning which the artist wished to portray, remains part of the manifest content. Venus has obviously overcome Mars, she has beaten him sexually; he is exhausted, she is cool. It represents the triumph of love over war (hate), good over evil, peace over strife; in fact, the theme is 'love conquers all'.

This was a brilliant theme because art historians tell us that this painting was commissioned by the Medici family as a wedding present to a male member of the Vespucci family, a connection to which Botticelli alluded by painting three little wasps in the foliage. 'Wasp' is *vespa* in Italian, a synonym of the Vespucci family.

So far, then, the manifest content of this work of art has been quite subtle, and there may be many more nuances in this picture which were only manifest to the Florentine families of the day.

But what about the painter? What do we know about Botticelli that may have influenced his choice of theme and subject?

First of all, this was a very daring painting in so far as it was one of the first in the developing school of secular art starting up in Florence at the end of the fifteenth century. Previously, art patrons had been associated with the Church and their commissions were all religiously orientated. This painting represents a pagan myth. Nevertheless, it may be that Botticelli could not quite overcome his religious convictions, and in choosing a pagan myth softened the blow by suggesting a Christian allegory in the Deposition of Christ. There is no doubt that it could be argued that the face of Venus could be interpreted as a tragic mask, and that her fingers signalled the Christian 'V' symbol, as do those of Mars, but to a less obvious degree. Mars himself is painted almost in the form of a deposed body rather than in living sleep and his lance, pointed more or less in the direction of his chest, is in a way reminiscent of the Roman centurion's spear. All this Christian symbolism would not have been lost to an inquisitive clergy and most likely exonerated Botticelli in their eyes. Nevertheless, it must be considered as yet another example of the painting's manifest content, albeit beautifully disguised.

However, in Florence also at this time the Neoplatonist philosophy was rapidly becoming widely discussed and gaining approval among the more secular elements of society, which included the artists and writers of the day. Botticelli was considered one of these and his paintings started to reflect this philosophy.

Neoplatonism was challenged by the monk Savonarola, whose return to fundamentalism was a sad regression in Renaissance history. Unfortunately, Botticelli was one who fell under Savonarola's influence, and in the last years of his life the painter destroyed several of his later works in fits of religious retribution for his secular sins.

I think that, if we are to look for a latent content in *Venus and Mars*, it is the signs of a developing unwillingness of the emotional hemisphere to continue to accept the logical left hemisphere's attraction to Neoplatonism – a moral conflict beautifully illustrated in non-verbal terms. It heralded an appalling ending to Botticelli's life in which the painter lost his will to paint and, in a terrifying

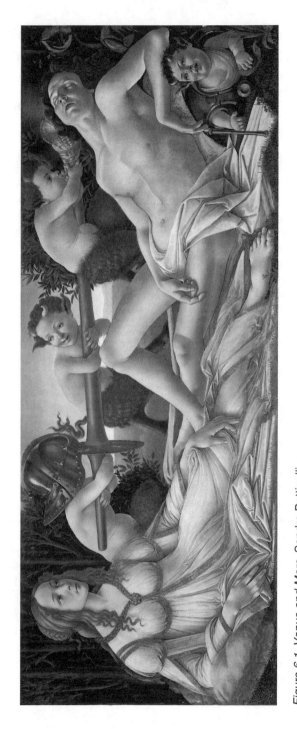

Figure 6.1 *Venus and Mars*, Sandro Botticelli
Source: By permission of the National Gallery, London.

attempt at atonement, sacrificed the very paintings in his possession. This conveniently introduces the theme of the use of art form in therapy.

THE USE OF ART FORM IN THERAPY

In the disposal of guilt

Cameral analysis encourages the patient to fashion an art form image of his problem and imbue it with any sin of which the patient feels guilty. Then by symbolically destroying this image the conflict it represented is no longer there. It is to be hoped that any associated symptoms will be resolved. It is interesting to speculate how this method would have fared in Botticelli's case. Once the problem became clear to the analyst the treatment could have involved the sacrifice of one painting, perhaps a painting commissioned by the analyst; by resolving the conflict, Botticelli's enthusiasm as an artist could have been restored and perhaps more of his work would have survived.

By utilizing the associated emotion when creating a work of art

Most of us will have witnessed the almost hysterical outflow of laughter from children daubing wet sand on one another by the edge of the sea, or slapping paint over a sheet of paper. In most modern art exhibitions there will be a vast canvas which looks as if the artist has literally slung buckets of paint at the surface from some distance away; their titles are often perplexing. Whichever way one looks at such creations one thing is certain: like the children, they must have been accompanied by much outpouring of emotion!

The creation of art form can have an affect on the artist similar to that of abreaction. By revealing conscious or unconscious fears and fantasies to external scrutiny, the creative act is the pictorial equivalent of a confession with all its cathartic values. Like abreaction, the art form re-creates the causal problem and allows it to surface for discussion, inspection and re-framing.

It is almost impossible to imagine the pain, discomfort and sheer physical exertion suffered by the aged Michelangelo in painting the vault of the Sistine Chapel. For four years, alone, lying on his back high up in the scaffolding, he could only have tolerated the task by the presence of an emotional 'high' sustained by the creative process, a creative process mirrored in one of the greatest miracles of art – his *Creation of Adam*.

In his poems, Michelangelo expressed anxiety about his work and felt that it could be deemed sinful. One can only guess that this was connected with his fascination for the male body, just as one can only surmise that his inspired effort in the Sistine Chapel was motivated by a desire for atonement of his imaginary sins. He even depicts himself in the ranks of the unrighteous being dragged down to hell in *The Last Judgement*.

In what better place could his right hemisphere confession be 'heard'?

Leaving aside for a moment artists themselves, art appreciation by others can generate strong emotions, and the more powerfully the art form is expressed the greater the influence on the viewer. An old medieval worshipper kneeling at the altar in the church of Santa Maria dei Frari in Venice and looking up at Titian's *Assumption of the Virgin* must have been greatly calmed and comforted from the anxieties of approaching death by the confidence and the certainty with which the promise of an after-life is portrayed.

Perhaps the most obvious way in which pent-up emotions, conscious or unconscious, can be expressed is through eroticism in art form. From the crude male and female genitalia displayed in the form of grafitti in men's and women's lavatories, through the more constructed nudes in the style of Picasso, to the refined sensuality of, say, Correggio's *Leda and the Swan*, all represent basic emotions calling for an outlet. Without such an outlet the danger of their repression might contribute to, or initiate, neurotic behaviour. Bacchanalian orgies, homosexuality, bestiality, masochism and sadism are constant art themes recurring throughout history, and have served as a cathartic function for every known civilization.

By making therapeutic use of art form which has been supposedly endowed with a supernatural force

The origin of the belief that an inanimate representation of a living creature can itself possess that creature's powers goes back over

20,000 years to palaeolithic times, according to Professor J.D. Lewis-Williams.

As director of the Rock Art Research Unit in the Department of Archaeology of the University of Witwatersrand, Professor Lewis-Williams considers that the European cave paintings of Lascaux and Altamira among others, were probably drawn by individuals having a tribal position similar to that of a shaman today. From his research into the lives of the southern San shamans of South Africa he showed that these people had for thousands of years similarly drawn and painted animal forms on cave walls. He is also of the opinion that these cave paintings were drawn while the artist was in an altered state of consciousness brought about by the sensory deprivation experienced in these caves. Professor Lewis-Williams has constructed a neurophysiological model of the ways in which mental imagery is perceived in certain altered states of consciousness, which involves the examination of entoptic (from the Greek *'ent'* and *'optic'*, meaning 'within vision') phenomena.[1]

The interesting theory arising out of this work is that the paintings were not merely decorative nor necessarily for instructive purposes but contained a powerful potency, such as strength and cunning equivalent to the animal depicted. In South Africa, within living memory, ancient cave paintings have been considered able to pass on this power to individuals (almost always shamans) who touch them while performing ritual, trance-inducing dances. The power these individuals were then considered to possess could be used for healing purposes. The caves themselves became very powerful places, similar to our own medieval cathedrals.

Dr Louise Oliver[2] of the Adult Guidance Institute, Pretoria, has studied the trance technique of the traditional African healer (a Malopo doctor, one who calls up the spirits causing the disease in the patient in an attempt to rid the patient of them) and considers that the altered state of consciousness that occurs while they are dancing in the Malopo ritual has the same external signs as the hypnotic trance. In this trance state the body is supposedly possessed by a spirit of one of either his or her own ancestors, or an alien spirit which may be animal in origin. This spirit then guides them in their divining and healing.

Illness amongst these primitive tribes is considered to be the result of deliberate invisible supernatural actions of malevolent beings and creatures, and it is to the supernatural they look to help in counteracting these actions.

Although Dr Oliver's research does not illustrate the involvement of art form it does confirm (1) the primitive belief that the human body can absorb an external spirit; (2) that the power of this spirit can be used therapeutically; and (3) that this so-called power appears to be a function of the right hemisphere in so far as it presents itself when the individual is in an hypnotic state.

Let us now return to art form and consider idolatry.

The belief that art form in the shape of an idol can carry the same power as the image it depicts is well known. The sacred carved stone gods in the temples of the Pharaohs, the sculptured images of the Olympian gods housed in Greek temples from Ephesus to Athens, the Roman Pantheon, the Christian Cross, totemism, the list is endless. All these images were considered to have healing powers, some more specifically than others. The Greek god Aesculapius was one such idol. In the Greek hospitals (*Aesculapii*) it was the custom to place, at the foot of his statue in his temple, small carvings of that part of the body which needed healing. This custom was carried on into Christianity. Offerings, fashioned from silver or gold, of the human anatomy, are still placed around the icon of the Virgin Mary in the church of Panaghia Evangelistria on the Greek island of Tinos (and other churches in Greece), in the belief that they will effect a cure of that diseased part in the sufferer.

An icon, a religious painting, a sacred relic, water from a sacred well or the River Jordan are all *tangible* objects, and *touching* them is a positive body sensation. If to this is added a positive (powerful) suggestion (belief) that the sensation perceived is in fact the god's healing touch, an immediate psychosomatic relief from the *anxiety* of illness is triggered off in the patient.

In the same way a talisman can be a great comfort, and its power depends on its owner's degree of belief in it. A patient of mine has several gold, silver and decorated crosses which can be worn as necklaces. The one she most values is a rather cheap, insignificant wooden cross she bought from a tourist stall outside the Vatican. This is the one she held up in her hand for the Pope to bless at a public audience in the auditorium next to St Peter's in Rome.

This belief in a talisman is instilled into the individual by suggestion, and can be as mundane as a lucky penny or a four-leaved clover, but whatever form the inanimate object takes, it is what it represents in the mind of the possessor that can determine a therapeutic value. It is perfectly possible, for instance, to take an object such as a ring and, under hypnosis, endow it with a belief.

A patient of mine, whom I shall call Paul, gradually developed a fear of flying which eventually became an unacceptable influence on his work. He was a businessman, and his work entailed occasional flurries of trips abroad. These trips were usually of an urgent nature and demanded the use of air transport rather than going by sea and train or car. He had never enjoyed flying, but a large gin was usually sufficient to get him aboard the aircraft where he was able to bury himself in some form of reading matter. Even so, if a foreign visit appeared to be on the horizon he would try to so organize it in advance that he could fit it in with a holiday, take his time and avoid flying.

Unfortunately, as business expanded, so did the necessity for him to travel abroad more frequently, and his coping method became less effective. He soon realized that he was becoming a much more nervous individual than he had been in the past. His wife noticed this change and at first put it down to pressure at work, but it was not until he started smoking again after a five-year abstinence that she realized that his problem was becoming serious, and demanded that he seek help. Tranquillizers were prescribed and were most effective. He stopped smoking and his *joie de vivre* returned. Then it happened. On a flight to Rome he panicked on board the aeroplane and had to be isolated and sedated by the cabin crew. He blamed his loss of control on the fact that he had taken more pills than he should have done, and he felt confused.

It is often very difficult, confronted with a case history such as this, to decide whether the basic problem was an underlying anxiety neurosis in the form of an agoraphobia and exacerbated by flying, or whether it was an isolated condition – a true flying phobia.

I think that some phobias, such as snake- and spider-phobias, are so universal that they could be considered as patterns of behaviour genetically transmitted. If this is true, then it is not unreasonable to consider such phobias as isolated mental phenomena. In this country they have a nuisance value, just as a deformed big toe may be annoying on occasions, but do not on the whole interfere with the quality of life and do not warrant any deep analytic treatment.

The majority of flying phobias can be placed in this category, and most of them can be successfully contained by the use of appropriate drugs. There is no need for deep and lengthy analyses in patients who are obviously well adjusted and in complete control of themselves in every other walk of life. I found no real evidence in Paul's past history to suggest an underlying anxiety state and felt that treatment targeted at his fear of flying would be sufficient.

In the course of taking Paul's history I had discovered that one of the highlights of his early childhood were his visits to his grandparents, who lived in the Southampton area. His grandmother had arthritis in her hip-joints and could not walk very far, but Paul loved her cooking. On the other hand, his grandfather, a retired schoolmaster, enjoyed walking, and especially if he had a companion such as his grandson. Their walks were always planned to include something interesting; how sailing boats sailed, how cranes could lift heavy weights, the difference between diesel and petrol engines, as well as why certain plants grew in certain soils. Back after the walk they would both go through it all again in front of Granny, explaining everything as if she were totally ignorant of the outside world!

Paul well remembers one occasion when, after excitedly explaining something to Granny, he turned to her, and in a very serious tone of voice, said, 'Grandpa knows *everything*, you know'. She surprised him by turning away and walking towards the kitchen blowing her nose, but not before Paul had noticed that there were tears in her eyes.

When his grandfather died he left Paul his gold hunter pocket-watch and his signet ring. I noticed he was wearing neither of these objects and asked him if he ever did so. He replied that he never wore a waistcoat and that, anyway, the watch had now become far too valuable. As for the ring, it was too loose and he was afraid of losing it but he did wear it on occasions with a dinner-jacket.

In treating Paul's flying phobia I employed my usual method of going through a typical flight sequence with the patient in hypnosis. During this sequence the patient was to experience nothing but a feeling of calmness as if it were a normal, everyday occurrence no different from taking the train to work. The suggestion was then given that this feeling of calmness would be present on any future occasion when an air flight was involved.

Combined with this was an explanation given, with the patient under hypnosis, of the irrationality of losing emotional control while in an aircraft, along with the reassurance of the statistical evidence confirming the recognized safety of air travel.

In addition, under hypnosis, I made the suggestion that were he to wear his grandfather's signet ring whenever he was to travel by air he would find that the very presence of the ring would remind him of the wisdom of his grandfather and this thought itself would be translated into a feeling of calmness and confidence. Furthermore, were any in-flight anxiety to develop, touching or twisting the ring would be such a comforting feeling that fear would be subdued.

Some weeks after his treatment I received a picture postcard from Singapore. It said: 'Remarkable! Thanks to Grandpa I almost enjoyed the flight! Paul.'

My secretary, who had obviously read the postcard, took it to be referring to me, and remarked that although she knew I was getting older she felt that Paul's description was 'a bit unfair'. I did not enlighten her.

Chapter 7

Cameral analysis and music and dance

Neurophysiological experiments have shown that the right hemisphere of the human brain is the main arbiter involved in music processing, although for one of the components, namely rhythm, the left hemisphere is equally efficient.

This is what one would expect from the different cognitive working processes employed by the two hemispheres. The temporal analytical method of the left hemisphere is well suited to the analysis of the linear repetition of rhythm but that is all. The right hemisphere, by spatially synthesizing the other components of music (including rhythm), such as timbre, harmony, pitch, intonation, resonance, melody and so on, is able to interpret them together so that they are perceived holistically as a musical composition.[1,2,3]

However, it is interesting to note that trained musicians who have had education in reading music and playing a musical instrument radically alter the pattern of hemispheric processing to include more left hemisphere participation.[4,5] Again, this finding can be explained if one considers that, in the educative process, the left hemisphere's analytical strategy was used to process a tune note by note, as in reading a book. One reads the symbols of a score just as one reads the letters of a word, a process which involves the left hemisphere.[6]

If, as neurophysiology suggests, music is intimately involved with the right hemisphere, then it becomes another method by which this hemisphere can express itself; by the same token it can be used as a two-way communication just like any other art form and therefore opens up the prospect of therapy involving music. Cameral analysis, with its capacity of direct communication with the right hemisphere by the use of hypnosis, is ideally suited to this form of therapy.

The world is full of noises, from the massive clap of thunder to the delicate song of the nightingale. Just as the use of sound has been developed by the nightingale to help in species preservation, so in humans, from the cradle lullaby to the sombre dead march, music has been used throughout our history to explain our purpose, express our joys and comfort our sorrows.

The late Professor N. Shipkowensky of Sophia University, writing in the book *Music and the Brain* (1977),[7] points out the universality of the use of music in the healing process. He first describes the use of music among primitive tribes and how songs were thought to have a supernatural origin, deriving from dreams or visions; how their healers, while in 'bizarre states of altered consciousness', drew on the use of music as an essential part of their curative practice.[8,9] Thus, by adding music, he echoes the primitive art theories of Professor Lewis-Williams and the observations of Dr Oliver and others in this field. Shipkowensky then goes on to trace the influence of Orphism from its Thracian origin, through the Greek and Roman worlds (quoting Bruno Meinecke's[10] assertion that 'psychiatric cases of various types were treated by song'), to the mental hospitals of Islam in the ninth to the twelfth centuries where music was reintroduced as a therapeutic process.[11] He is sadly of the opinion that the curative power of music has been mistakenly ignored by present-day psychiatrists.

Shipkowensky recognises five basic varieties of musical therapy: background, contemplative, combined, performing and creative. It is in the 'combined' classification that he relates the induction, maintenance and termination of hypnosis with the simultaneous playing of music. He gives due credit to Anton Mesmer as the first to practise this approach, and points out the importance of his combining *suggestion* with the music.

I use music in Mode Two of the cameral analytical method; that is, of course, with the patient in hypnosis. It is used:

1 As a method for deepening the hypnotic state. Almost any soothing sort of music will suffice – music not necessarily known to the patient. I prefer classical piano music, such as Chopin's nocturnes.
2 As an aid in age regression when favourite tunes of yesteryear are played to the patient in order to enhance important memor-

ies of that particular period in their lives. This is fairly generalized, rather in the style of *Pennies from Heaven*, as per Potter.
For instance, *La Mer*, to one of my patients, took her back to
the tragic death of her wartime fiancé, and was very helpful in
abreacting the emotion associated with his death, something
she needed to mourn but which had been denied her at the
time.

3 The use of a *specific* tune to abreact emotions associated with
   the underlying problem. I can instance many of these, but as an
   example the school hymn was a very powerful adjunct to the
   memory of bullying and homosexual practices forced on a
   patient of mine when he was a boarder at his public school.

4 As a powerful method of communicating ideas and suggestions
   of a therapeutic nature along with the re-educative exposure of
   symptoms. For example, with the patient in hypnosis one can
   play music and accompany it with suggestions of well-being,
   growing confidence, peace and tranquillity – in fact, incorporate
   an ego-strengthening regime. Alternatively, one can ask the
   patient to provide a tape or a record of their own favourite
   music and use this to the accompaniment of re-educative and
   re-constructing suggestions. The type of music should fit the
   character of the patient as well as being in tune with the nature
   of the suggestions.

In my opinion music, as a mainly right hemisphere communication system, is only equalled by poesis, and it is interesting to
note that the late Professor John Blacking of Queen's University
(Belfast) maintained that music was an important means of communication across all cultural boundaries and that the study of
ethnomusicology could influence the integration of an immigrant
population into its host country. In America, jazz, soul and blues
music has told the story of the initially enslaved people's struggle
for identity, in an emotional manner and with a poignancy that no
verbal form of communication could ever hope to achieve. It is a
pity that the Western approach to music is so elitist that it discour-
ages its potential and thus denies a lot of its value in interethnic
understanding.

Music combined with rhythmical body movement can induce an
altered state of consciousness in which therapeutic emotional cath-
arses can take place.

It is very easy to see the vastness of emotional release in the tribal dancing of primitive races, when most of the participants end up in states of total exhaustion. It is not difficult to observe similar states in basic Western dancing where music combined with a strong beat has created such energetic displays as rock-and-roll, jive and so on, and more recently slam-dancing. The sudden liberation of sexual behaviour with the advent of the contraceptive pill in the 1960s has brought with it teenage social stresses with which many find difficulty in coping. Musically induced emotional releases witnessed in 'gigs' are one way of resolving stress and can be considered as an effective and harmless therapeutic throwback. But there is a danger.

In primitive tribes the emotional release and its accompanying high state of suggestibility is under the control of tribal elders and their medicine-men. They make sure it is devils that are cast out and only friendly spirits called in.

Unfortunately, acid house parties, all-night raves, gigs and so forth have no such controlling factor. Instead, circling the herd like beasts of prey are the drug-pushers offering alternative methods of stress therapy. They know where to find their victims, who, because they are in this high state of suggestibility, easily succumb to their fatal attraction. In Western society the more basic forms of music and dance can often open the door to devilish 'spirits' simply because the emotional needs of the right hemisphere have been ignored by a society failing to educate its youth into coping with these needs. These spirits, like the Seven Dwarfs, have wonderful names – speed, acid, grass, dope, hash, smack and coke – but the lives of the Snow Whites who rejoice in their Dantesque company never have a happy ending.

The therapeutic value of music lies in its ability to conjure up emotions from ecstasy to melancholy as well as physically to express (release) them in song and dance. As in primitive tribes, a controlled form of mass therapy could be introduced to present-day group therapy on Shipkowensky's lines.

I am indebted to Dr Dabney Ewin for drawing my attention to just such a method developed by a Brazilian psychiatrist, Dr David Akstein of Rio de Janeiro. Dr Akstein has made a lengthy study of ritual 'kinetic trances', which form part of the culture of various Afro-Brazilian sects as well as European and Middle Eastern subcultures such as the whirling dervishes of Turkey and Egypt. In coining the phrase 'kinetic trance', Akstein defines it as an hypnotic state induced through musically accompanied bodily movements (mostly rotational), with the head held in an unnatural position.

These ritual kinetic trances, by the profound release of tensions, have strong therapeutic affects on their followers, and Akstein goes on to observe that millions of individuals, belonging to such Brazilian spiritualist sects as the Umbanda, Candomble and Quimbanda, find in them a means of escape from their daily worries, a release of pent-up emotions, and a resulting psychic and psychosomatic equilibrium.

From these observations Akstein has developed a form of *non-verbal* group psychotherapy which he has called Terpsichorean Trance Therapy (TTT), in which the hypnotic state is induced and maintained by music and dance-movement.[12] He is at pains, however, to emphasize that all spiritualism, possession states, mysticism, religious rituals and so on play no part whatsoever in either the induction or maintenance of TTT's kinetic trance; the whole activity takes place within a strict medical framework, the controller being a fully qualified psychotherapist, and each patient has a personal controller.

Akstein is a psychiatrist and employs conventional psychiatic methods in treating his patients. In his clinic he discusses the patient's problems in the usual way, giving support therapy and medication where necessary. He will also resort to special techniques if deemed desirable, such as hypnosis or other forms of relaxation. TTT is one of his special techniques but is essentially a group therapy involving the social class setting to which the patient is accustomed, and over the years he has perfected a routine which he feels produces the best results.

What follows is a brief description of TTT, along with a few comments of my own relating to cameral analysis and hemispheric asymmetry. TTT meetings are held once a week and each session lasts 45 minutes. An informal environment is encouraged, with dimmed lights, loose comfortable clothing, light shoes or bare feet and plenty of room in which to move around.

New patients have been briefed on the method and its objectives but no pattern of behaviour is suggested or demanded from the patient.

Immediately before and after the session a record is made of such clinical data as blood-pressure, pulse-rate and so forth, and, on a separate form, details of the trance characteristics such as

depth, intensivity of movements, time distortion, sensory disturbances and amnesia for future reference.

Akstein divides the treatment under hypnosis into two phases.
In the first phase each operator stands in front of the patient and
asks him to close his eyes and concentrate on overcoming his
problem. He then asks the patient to breathe deeply (hyperventi-
late) and, as he does so, rythmic, drum-beat music is played, which
will continue throughout the session.

About 1 minute after beginning hyperventilation, the operator
leads the patient into a counter-clockwise rotational movement
of the whole body; while doing so the patient either bends forward with his chin close to his chest or bends backwards with
his face upwards. In this first phase, which is considered to be
a phase of desensitization, the kinetic trance induced tends
to be more frenetic and demands a close control by the operator's
assistant.

Gradually, the patient's movements slow, and he enters the
second, or re-structuring, phase. It is at this point that the music is
changed to a more melodious (but still rhythmical) style and the
operator (or his assistant) steadies the patient's balance and induces him to dance to the rhythm of the music.

Akstein maintains that musical scores, even very short ones, can
elicit memories, association of ideas, problem solving, creativity
and regression. In so doing they facilitate the re-structuring of the
personality.[13]

When the patient is finally balanced and holding pace with the
music he is left entirely on his own; in doing so he chooses his own
mode of behaviour.

From the onset of the music to the end of the session no verbal
communication with the patient takes place.

The session is terminated by fading out the music and slow
inhibition of the dancers by their operators, who, at the same time,
verbally encourage their patient to open their eyes and return to
their normal state of consciousness.

There are several interesting neurophysiological points to observe in Akstein's method. Three of these can be seen in the
induction of his kinetic trance state by non-verbal procedures, the
first of which is his use of hyperventilation. Hyperventilation is, in
itself, well recognised as a non-verbal method of hypnotic induction,[14] and its introduction just prior to the drum-beat must give an
added impetus to the onset of the kinetic trance. The neurological

explanation of its mode of action lies in the diminution of plasma carbon-dioxide (PCO_2) washed out with the over-breathing, thus producing a respiratory alkalosis.

It has been shown (Lum 1981)[15] that there is an initial marked *increase* in neuronal activity as a result of quite *minor* falls in plasma CO_2. (If, however, hyperventilation continues there is produced a neuronal *depression* which, if allowed to continue, progresses to tetany, stupor and coma.) One of the effects of this initial increase is to stimulate the brain-stem reticular formation and, as explained in Chapter 2, the inhibiting function of this structure reduces global awareness,[16] which powerfully aids the induction of hypnosis.

I should mention at this point that, apart from its role in hypnotic induction, hypocarbia has been incriminated in functional illness, particularly anxiety states.

Many physicians recognize a 'hyperventilation syndrome,'[17] which seems to be a common affliction of sedentary town-dwellers who are chronic and habitual hyperventilators (over-breathers). These patients often present with a variety of functional symptoms, and treatment methods solely concerned with the re-education of their breathing habits have been surprisingly successful according to Dr L.C. Lum, a chest physician of Papworth Hospital in Cambridge, who claims a 75 per cent cure rate after twelve months.[18]

The second interesting point is Akstein's use of rhythm.

I have previously drawn attention to the work of Gruzelier and Brow (1984),[19] who considered that the prerequisite of hypnotic induction is an initial left hemisphere bias and subsequent left hemisphere inhibition. Akstein substitutes the voice of the hypnotist (which is interpreted by the patient's verbal, left hemisphere) with the monotonous rhythm of the drum-beat, which has also been shown to be a left hemisphere interpretive task.[20] By *commencing* the session with the drum-beat, it is thus the left hemisphere that is initially activated, reducing its global awareness to a single auditory stimulus. This in effect inhibits this hemisphere, leaving the right hemisphere to interpret the later, and more melodious, music symbols in the emotional body-language of dance-form.

Third, the anticlockwise rotation of the body, along with what Akstein terms 'the antinatural posture' of the trunk and head, produces a strong excitation of the vestibular apparatus in its function as a regulator of balance. This high, sub-cortical stimulus (according to Asktein) induces an inhibitory cortical reaction favouring trance formation (cf. hypocarbia).

Finally, TTT has been designed as a group-therapy treatment. Why?

It appears to me that Asktein, in his detailed research into possessional states, has identified a powerful therapeutic force in group participation. Although each patient has an individual therapist to observe and, if necessary, to control his or her emotional releases, he or she must be aware of the other patients (probably by means of the 'hidden observer' phenomenon) in a similar kinetic trance state.

It could be that this 'awareness' is the source of the added impact, just as group prayer, mass ritual behaviour, chanting in chorus, can produce heightened emotional reactions in a susceptible gathering (that is, a gathering of individuals with a specific belief).

Where cameral analysis is concerned, the use of music in treatment, compared with TTT, is less energetic and constitutes a combined therapy as previously outlined in the four groups:

1 as a method of deepening the hypnotic state;
2 as an aid to age regression;
3 to encourage an abreaction;
4 to reinforce therapeutic suggestions along with re-educative symptom exposure.

(In the re-educative process the property of music to sublimate baser emotions into a higher, more socially acceptable level is fully exploited.)

Chapter 8

Cameral analysis and poetry

I am two fooles, I know,
For loving, and for saying so
In whining Poetry;
But where's that wiseman, that would not be I,
If she would not deny?
Then as th'earths inward narrow crooked lanes
Do purge sea waters fretful salt away,
I thought, if I could draw my paines,
Through Rimes vexation, I should them allay,
Griefe brought to numbers cannot be so fierce,
For, he tames it, that fetters it in verse.

John Donne, 1571–1631: from *The Triple Foole*

POETRY AS A THERAPEUTIC FORCE

Poetry takes an emotion and clothes it in words. It becomes therefore an example of interhemispheric co-operation. But, more than that, poetry itself is a language with a combined lexicon of words and emotions *unique* to each poet.

The poem itself, *at its point of creation*, is a symbiotic expression of both hemispheres of the poet's mind. It represents, as it were, an interhemispheric solution frozen in time.

The solution – that is, the poem – implies a problem. The problem can be simply anything from an everyday irritation to deciding on a particular political stance or expressing a philosophy. But the solution is strictly a personal one and serves, at its point of creation, in maintaining the sanity of the poet.

Poets, especially good ones, are very complicated individuals often labelled by society from 'slightly off-beat' to 'distinctly eccentric'. I do not believe poets set out to be poets but find in poetry a method of surviving in a world, the faults of which they see clearly. Perhaps I should add: more clearly, and with more sensitivity than the rest of us.

This makes them vulnerable, and their work exposes their vulnerability.

Thomas Lovell Beddoes was a poet whose works showed a morbid fascination with death. He poisoned himself. Sylvia Plath is another, among many other poets, who committed suicide. This death list is morbidly long, but the list of the survivors is more comforting and, in my opinion, is a tribute to the therapeutic power of poetry in such company.

But although we are not all poets of this magnitude – and I would like to distinguish between a poet and someone writing a poem – we can use the same process in coming to terms with our difficulties whether this be in personal composition or with the help of analytical therapy.

The combined skills of the two hemispheres produce, in poetry, new powers in words by releasing their connotative and meta-phoric possibilities as opposed to the precise meanings usually demanded by the logical left hemisphere.

These connotations involve sound, as in assonance, meter, rhyme, alliteration, figures of speech such as puns on whole or even half words. Nothing is impossible, even nonsense words can convey an emotionally ordered, but nevertheless mad scene, as this from *Alice through the Looking-glass*:

> T'was brillig, and the slithy toves
> Did gyre and gimble in the wabe;
> All mimsy were the borogoves,
> And the mome raths outgrabe.

I believe that in poetry the hemispheres often poke fun at each other and enjoy the joke between themselves. In this next cleri-hew, for instance, I do not think it too far-fetched to imagine a smile coming over the left-hand side of the face as the right hemisphere points out the apparent absurdity of left hemisphere logic!

> If the man who turnips cries,
> Cry not when his father dies,

> 'Tis a proof that he had rather
> Have a turnip than his father.
> Samuel Johnson 1709–1784

Nor perhaps the smirk on the right-hand side of the face as the left hemisphere counters by demonstrating the inadequacy of sound alone to convey the subtleties of meaning.

Perhaps this is the origin of the wry smile?

Christopher Ricks, in his brilliant essay[1] on Beddoes, quotes the following:

> For death is more 'a jest' than Life, you see
> Contempt grows quick from familiarity.
> I owe this wisdom to Anatomy.

Ricks then goes on to explain:

> The taunting triplet depends not only on the nimble blasé way in which the familiar and contemptuous pun on 'quick' is bred, but also on Anatomy's being the subtle medical training as well as the unsubtle skeleton itself.[2]

One way, therefore, in which poetry acts as a therapeutic force is on the poet personally. As I have already suggested, the process of producing a poem involves an interhemispheric mechanism by which both hemispheres come to a mutual understanding of a problem. The poem becomes their own solution and has a therapeutic value to the poet in the form of a re-structuring process. So, purely from the poet's point of view, once the poem is completed the therapy has taken place, and although re-reading the poem at later dates may serve to reinforce the mental re-structuring, the poem's real value lay at the point of its creation.

This conception is taken much further by Murray Cox and Alice Theilgaard in their exciting and original book *Mutative Metaphors in Psychotherapy* (1987).[3] In this important work they describe a mode of dynamic psychotherapy in which two distinct processes are involved; they call it the 'Aeolian Mode'. These two processes are the 'dynamic components' and the 'therapeutic initiatives'. The dynamic components are three in number: poiesis; aesthetic imperatives; and points of urgency. But it is their definition of poiesis that mirrors the therapeutic influence I attribute to poetry.

Cox and Theilgaard use the term 'poiesis' as a dynamic part of creativity which takes place at the point at which a poem is on 'the brink of being called into being for the first time'. It is this cognitive/affective connotation that a therapist must be on 'perceptive tiptoe' to discern as it occurs.

They consider this new material, in whatever guise it appears, to be of great importance in both analytic and supportive psychotherapy, in that it has been freshly created in a mode *free from the inhibitive chains of past influences*.

It would be quite wrong of me, by taking poiesis out of context, to give such an isolated impression of one aspect of the Aeolian Mode. One thing above all that Cox and Theilgaard's book emphasizes is the *total presence*, the *holistic creativity*, of a patient being of paramount importance to psychotherapy. Like the patient, the book must be taken as a whole. The authors, showing a literary inspiration characteristic throughout the book, have taken a quotation from Bachelard[4] to illustrate their theme: '*But the image has touched the depths before it stirs the surface.*' They have drawn up from the depths the images and metaphors to form a theoretically original, therapeutically practical, co-ordinated work of immense interest to all of us in the medical profession.

Continuing on the theme of *the therapeutic value of a poem to the poet* himself, poetry, like other art forms, can be used:

1 as an analytical uncovering agent to help in exposing the roots of a problem;
2 as a therapeutic help in the mental re-framing of a problem in order to lessen the disrupting and incapacitating effect of any interhemispheric discrepancies.

As in dreams, a poem can be considered to have a manifest and latent content, but in the poem both are usually more obvious and interpretation more accurate.

Frequently a poem will give information which the poet has found difficult, either because of inhibition or plain embarrassment, to express in any other way.

The following poem gave me the first indication of my patient's anxiety concerning his fear of possible homosexuality. Although the Mode One analytical interview had revealed a past crisis of faith, a matter which had been freely discussed, I was still under the impression that, as a married man with children and possessing a healthy and normal sexual interest in women, the question of homosexuality did not arise.

He then presented me with this poem, which had been written, in an intentionally excessive style, at a time when he had been wrestling with various religions in an attempt to come to some sort of an answer as to what he, himself, could reasonably believe.

He had never shown this poem to any other person. In allowing me to read it he, almost nonchalantly, revealed to me the strong underlying problem of his homosexual fears and neatly opened up the subject for discussion.

It tells much more besides!

To single out one aspect of the poem: the Noble Eightfold Path of Buddhism, with its three constituents of moral self-discipline, meditation and wisdom, is almost inextricably intertwined with a form of sexual emotion the poet considers dangerous and of which he must be beware.

One could consider each to be logically separate arguments, but emotionally they become indivisible. *The poem, by bringing together the logical and the emotional, becomes an interhemispheric discussion document.*

At this stage the poem shows that both hemispheres are, at least, at one with a problem although the answer seems as far away as ever. Later in the patient's life he came to realize that his early feelings were a normal part of developing heterosexuality which, in his case, were occurring at a time when he was being actively pressurized into 'brotherly love'. Unfortunately, decisions made in this early period of anguish had a long-term effect on his life. It was problems arising from their affect (emotion) that needed an analytic resolution.

Aulie

> Never mind the dying forests, Aulie,
> Beware the passing show, the suffering breath.
> Rise like the moon from the sublunary.
> Phenomena are in cahoots with death.
>
> Beware the lavish stratagems of nature.
> Beware the hooking miracles of art.
> Put them behind you, swerving high and wide
> Towards elimination of the heart.
>
> Down on the coastline of the *richissimes*
> You cultivate detachment like a bridge,

Footing slow the Noble Eightfold Path
Along the litany of privilege;

Casting wide your window, stepping out
Into the holy metaphor of ocean;
Free to spend all day intuiting
The principles of spiritual motion;

Feeling the woods unbroken at your back,
Watching Narcissus cartwheel on the lawn
(More handsome than you care to recognize);
Speaking to none and being waited on.

The *Dhammapada* is your chosen text.
Far out, far out, you track the shining fins.
You meditate out on the balcony.
Narcissus, garden boy, looks up and grins.

You try so hard to live upon abstraction;
You sleep with transience – or so it seems.
You leave a silvery trail of slow success
Until Narcissus cartwheels through your dreams

And suddenly nature changes overnight
Into a yowl of sensuality –
The recent prayers of the snow-fed streams
Are chuckling proofs of your carnality.

The sea, once proxy for eternity,
Mimics the shifting border of desire.
The musky twilight, fingering the wall,
Spreads through the pines, aghast with sex and fire.

What do you do? You put muscle on your bones.
The bars and bells you keep beneath your bed
Burn daily in the white Atlantic light.
You stretch and sweat, the sacred books unread,

The jeremiads battling in your head,
Predictable, exactly violent.
(You do not see they only serve to mask
The stealthy progress of engorged intent.)

This love is love of love for the sake of love,
An injury of mirrors in the night,

A pushmipulyu wanted to be wanted,
An accident that obligates a flight.

All this you know. Now you must learn again.
Narcissus (garden boy) will be your lover.
And you will win and lose and lose again.
And sorrow in the dark when it is over.

A dozen impulses, the vernal wood,
A sense of doom on rising in the morning.
Moksha seems as far away as ever.
Fresh guano splatters on the awning.

When this patient came to me he was depressed, found very great difficulty in concentrating, and his mind was occupied with banal worries. At times he felt hypochondriacal and seemed obsessed with death. He felt he led a fraudulent existence, considered himself a failure and saw little point to his life.

Obviously, he was an individual with a serious unresolved problem or problems which were occupying most of his thinking time, leaving his conscious living bereft of logical continuity and sparse in initiative.

His poem discloses two (at least) separate emotional problems; a crisis of faith (in its wider sense), and an unresolved sexual anxiety. In the poem both problems are almost inextricably interwoven in a talent of metaphor and triple entendre reminiscent of Beddoes.

In my opinion this poem, at the time it was written, enabled the poet to identify, and by doing so, come to terms with, the presence of at least one unresolved anxiety. The poem had a delaying effect because it turned out to be just one of many onion-skins that had to be peeled off before he was able metaphorically to re-enter society with a freedom from guilt, invigorated and determined.

As in many of my patients, poetry played a varying therapeutic role. In some it had no value, in others it was useful in a very minor capacity. Often it was helpful in the re-educative re-structuring process, but whenever the patient was able to write poetry it was always of great advantage to the outcome of the therapy. The following is one such example.

Miss A was transferred to me by a colleague who had been treating her for 'problems of concentration and attention which interfered with her work'. When, in the course of her career, she moved into my area, he was anxious that she continue with treatment. She was 27 years old.

He felt that there was 'an underlying problem more extensive and characterological in nature', and went on to say, 'She evidences both anxiety and dysthymic features in a passive aggressive personality with strong depressive elements'. He ended his letter by saying that he felt she had 'serious psychological problems and was very much in need of continuous psychotherapy'.

To this I must add that she had difficulty sleeping, had bouts of uncontrollable crying, and felt tired and washed-out in the mornings. Her anger against society was most noticeable in her general conversation, which appeared guarded almost to the point of suspicion.

Probably a difficult case. Extraordinarily, it was quite the opposite, thanks to poetry.

Initially, I found her somewhat sullen; she was very disparaging of both herself and of the hypocrisy of the world around her. She exuded hate but was unable to explain these feelings; they appeared as a general bitterness as well as anger towards her own problem and the apparent inability of anyone to help her.

On the plus side she was obviously very intelligent, and when drawn out into conversation showed not only the command of a good vocabulary but the where-with-all to express it in terms which left nothing misunderstood.

I felt that somewhere along the line she had faced a period of severe rejection and her guarded cynicism was a protection from being hurt again. It was up to me to uncover the source of rejection and to re-frame it into love rather than hate.

In the course of Mode One analysis I had noted her fondness for music and poetry and brought them into therapy at the first opportunity. Even so, I was surprised at the sudden change in attitude poetry evoked.

I chose to introduce the concept of love (as opposed to hate) by a simple quote from Raymond Carver. I chose him because he epitomized the discovery of the value of love under extreme adversity. I read to her:

> And did you get what
>   you wanted from life, even so?
> *I did*.
> And what did you want?

> *To call myself beloved, to feel myself*
> *beloved on earth.*

I felt these words go home. She had not come across Carver before.

Miss A arrived early for her next appointment and in place of her usually apathetic stance she looked quite bright and smart. She was hardly seated before she blurted out how much she had enjoyed Carver. Since her last appointment she had read everthing that Carver had published, including his collections of short stories! The rest of the hour was spent discussing his work but, more importantly, how she herself related to it. It was very evident that she experienced his words emotionally, and had absorbed his purely right hemisphere message: to love the present rather than regret the past. I said a quiet word of thanks to Raymond Carver.

From this point onwards her progress was rapid. The most meaningful communication, both in and out of hypnosis, was through poetry. Her moods and feelings were almost always expressed in quotations. For instance, she gave me a paperback of Wallace Stevens in which small slips of pink sticky paper had been used to mark certain of his poems.

Most important of all were her own poems, the creation of which gave her a wonderful sense of relief and a growing confidence in herself as they were used in the re-structuring of her mental attitudes.

Here are two examples of them:

every morning
gertrude sings
a renewal
gertrude, the
proverbial
morning person

groaning in
evolution
as amphisbaena
crawls
out of pull-you
darkness
toward push-me
dawn
legless, four-eyed,

guilty
as the worm
splits
black theatre
of potential

four limbs, a
bitter taste,
erection

I brush my
teeth
ready to face
the world

My patient accompanied this poem with the following annotation:

Trying to portray daily awakening as an evolution and as a
moment where the cosmic, the sexual,
the banal meet.
will leave Gertrude Stein alone for now.
Amphisbaena (cosmic) ape [probably not developed enough]
(sexual)
human (banal and composite)
unconscious/dream/original sin/dawn of civilization/eternity and
conscious
movement into time (2 heads, split/extreme effort to say 'I will
live'/life in its activity, all colours,
power, macro-microcosm/→ awareness of
limbs, further differentiation, again, knowledge of good and
evil a bitter taste; mouth upon waking;
fellatio/sex as animalistic, involuntary urge primarily responsible for our erection on two feet;
getting out of bed an evolution i.e. from all fours to erect;
morning erection→ speaking subject
emerges as 'I' in carrying out the ordinary tasks of life; face of
an individual last body part/the
whole world within and without.

The second poem, with no comments:

having observed the frottage of a disco,
even as people pretend their pelvises

don't exist,
i conclude they wear pyjamas too, naked only
in their crapulence,
pathetic phallusies in two-four time.

my magniloquent hips, my callipygous form
conversed together, revelling within, the
site of sex,
(they speculate i want it, that i came for them
amidst the strobes)
i exit laughing, jouissance intact.

It is not my intention to reveal any details of the analysis of this case history; my object was merely to illustrate the use of poetry in cameral analysis. Suffice it to say within three months Miss A's whole demeanour had softened, she could concentrate well and was no longer depressed. Her sleep pattern was back to normal, she looked bright and alert, and she was pleased to notice that people who had previously appeared to avoid her were now seeking her friendship. A smile had replaced the scowl. At this point, her work done, she left my orbit.

Some two years later on a brief visit, she regaled, over coffee, her hopes and anxieties for the future. The intervening years had not been without problems, but the problems had not been insoluble. She had achieved distinction in her work and had found great comfort in her emotional life, which was about to be consummated by marriage. She had continued to write poetry. One group of poems were in celebration of her husband's birthday, poems which I would like to feel 'from loves awakened root do bud out now'. Here is one of them:

Your Effect

I should tell you when I begin to write
about you my inspiration backs up
like a seventy-two car pile-up
on the freeway of love and it is days
before the unceasing traffic flows smoothly again.

I should tell you when I begin to write
about you my throat feels like the ringed necks
of those African desert women:

heavy with a wealth of song, strangely regal,
but parched, parched with the merciless sun's heat.

I should tell you these things to avoid
romantic notions of a clear
and unimpeded lava flow
pouring out of my pen over
the edges of my desk out into the street.

I do acquire a rosy glow
in the ridiculous wrestle
with myself to acknowledge and
do justice to the difficult blessings
of abundance I have in you.

You, traffic cop in a hopeless jam.
You, gourd of water in a siccative landscape.
You, my fever and my cool relief.
You.

Miss A, I predict, will become a poet of our time.

Her poems invariably show a clear insight into muddled philoso-
phies, Nature's anomalies, or contentious human beliefs, which
she feels she needs to highlight *in her own mind* in order to live
with their absurdity. Poetry more powerfully illuminates a theme
than mere words, and these poems could be of great value to
others who, like herself, find difficulty at times in coming to terms
with life's variance. She must continue to write poetry, and, it is to
be hoped, publish it in the near future!

Chapter 9

Multiple personality syndrome

Dr Ferenc Völgyesi, in his book *Hypnosis of Man and Animals* (1966),[1] quotes from the work of Paracelsus (the seventeenth-century philosopher and physician)[2] what appears to be the first recorded history of a case of multiple personality. Völgyesi's description of this case is as follows:

> The hostess of a tavern near Basel had accused her servants for many months of stealing the daily takings. One day she found blood on her bedclothes and on the table, where there were also pieces of broken glass. It then came out that her 'second self' as a sleepwalker pilfered her own money which her 'original self' later found intact, hidden away in the roof. The 'original self' remembered nothing of this activity.

In the annals of medicine since Paracelsus many case histories of multiple personality have been published; these were particularly rife in the nineteenth century. The famous physician Weir Mitchell wrote about Mary Reynolds.[3] Pierre Janet described an anorectic patient, Marceline, who converted to normal eating after suggestion under hypnosis but unfortunately kept reverting to her anorectic state after only a few weeks of normalcy. In her anorectic state she had no knowledge of her periods of normality. William James and Max Dessoir were others of note who found hypnosis of value in the treatment of their multiple personality patients.

In an earlier chapter in this book on the history of hemispheric laterality I mentioned one such nineteenth-century case history of a dual personality, Felida X.[4] This patient, who was first seen in 1858 by a French physician, Dr Azam, was brought to the attention of the British medical profession by the Cambridge don Frederick Myers. Myers, in describing the two personalities of

Felida X, suggested that hypnosis could re-arrange the looms of her mind into a single, normally functioning pattern.

Some years ago (in 1978) I was present at a meeting in the Royal Society of Medicine (London) in which a similar case of dual personality was presented by Dr Gilbert Maher-Loughnan, a consultant physician working at the Colindale and Brompton hospitals.

This young woman was a true somnambulist; that is, in lay terms, she was a sleep-walker. Unfortunately, in her sleep-walking she was also an arsonist and set fire to rooms in her own home as well as buildings some distance away from her home. Until someone caught her in the act she was totally unaware of this side of her life and even then, in her waking state, had no recall of her activities while asleep. Dr Maher-Loughnan was able to produce total recall under hypnosis, and suggested that she would also remember all the events in the normal waking state. His treatment was completely successful; a fact that was confirmed by the patient herself who was present at the reading of Maher-Loughnan's paper and who very willingly answered searching questions from the audience after the paper had been given. In the three years that had passed since the termination of her treatment her somnambulistic habits had completely ceased, she had become more calm in herself and led a happier and more fulfilling life. As Myers had predicted, Dr Maher-Loughnan had been able to 're-arrange the looms of the [her] mind'.

From my point of view, however, this case also showed that the altered state of consciousness in which her arsonist activities took place was

1 a state of apparently full awareness in that she was able to dress normally and find her way about the town without causing any undue comment;
2 a state in which she was able to perform successful acts of arson without any apparent moral qualm;
3 one in which she had complete amnesia of these complicated events in her waking state and yet had *complete recall under hypnosis*.

If, then, under hypnosis this patient could achieve total recall of her somnambulistic activities, it is not unreasonable to assume that these activities were carried out while the patient was functioning in a similar state of altered consciousness to that of hypnosis. If, as has been suggested, this altered state of consciousness is a right hemisphere function, it would follow that this patient's problem had its origin in this hemisphere. However, before assuming this conjecture, let us consider the fact that this apparently 'normal' young woman exhibited a pathological inability to recall verbally major events and activities physically performed while in this state. In other words, there appears to be a serious memory loss in the so-called 'waking state', and yet we know that this is only an *apparent* memory loss because of the ability to remember the events under hypnosis. What must be considered is that this complete loss of knowledge occurring in the waking verbal state is very similar indeed to the findings from investigations into the memory and behaviour of Roger Sperry's split-brained patients. But these patients are anatomically abnormal, whereas we know that Dr Maher-Loughnan's patient was not. It would appear that a non-damaged brain (our normal self) is capable of producing a state of brain-function similar to that produced when the inter-hemispheric connections of the corpus callosum are severed. We know this to be neurologically feasible through the inhibitory potentials of the reticular formation.

To illustrate another important aspect of the multiple personality syndrome I would like to refer back to a well-documented nineteenth-century case history recorded under the pseudonym of 'Louis V'.

From my point of view this case stands out with particular importance in so far as this patient's personalities were accompanied by hysterical paralyses of parts of his body. The paralysed parts differed according to which 'personality' was dominant but were specific to that personality and a constant part of it. Moreover, as most of his life was spent in medical or mental institutions, a very accurate medical description of his life history was (and still is) available.

One of the many physicians in charge of Louis V during his lifetime was Dr M.J. Voisin, who published his findings in the French *Archive de Neurologie* in 1885, but an English review of the implications of this case was published in 1886 by Dr A.T. Myers, a relative, I believe, of the Cambridge don F.W. Myers (of Felida X fame). What follows is a précis of this patient's medical history as given in Dr Myers's paper.

Born in Paris in 1863, Louis V was the illegitimate child of a woman known to be of a bad character. As is so often discovered in cases of multiple personality, Louis V was severely ill-treated as a child, and in this case it was his mother who ill-treated him.

Louis V was convicted of theft at the age of ten and sentenced to remand in the reformatory of Saint Urbain for the next seven years. Here he obtained a primary education, which he had previously lacked. He was rarely out of one institution or another for the rest of his life.

At the age of fourteen, while working in the fields at Saint Urbain, he was suddenly terrified by a viper winding itself round his arm. That evening he developed an hysterical paraplegia with paralysis of both legs.

Three years later, and still paralysed, he was transferred to Bonneval Asylum, where he was given work as a tailor. Six months after his arrival at Bonneval he threw what was described as an hystero-epileptiform attack, from which he emerged free from all paralysis and believing he was back in the fields at Saint Urbain.

He had no knowledge whatsoever of his life since the viper incident, a matter of some three-and-a-half years.

His character while paralysed in both legs had been one of quiet co-operation, industrious and orderly. With the return of his non-paralysed state he became quarrelsome, greedy, violent, and he started stealing again.

Dr Camuset, in whose care he was at Bonneval, concluded that Louis V was a case of dual personality similar to Felida X. He was discharged from Bonneval, with full faculties, at the age of eighteen.

The next important point in his medical history was his admission to Bicêtre Hospital some two years later, following a conviction for theft. Here he came under the jurisdiction of Dr Voisin. Five months after his admission to this hospital he had an attack, described by Dr Voisin as 'hystero-epilepsy', which ended with a paralysis. This time the paralysis was in the form of a right hemiplegia, and his memory was a curious mixture of parts of his life but his habits were quiet and orderly, similar to those during his paralysed state following the viper incident.

Dr Voisin found his patient fascinating, and gives a full account of Louis V's medical history at Bicêtre, which included the use of hypnosis. Under hypnosis, his right-sided hysterical paralysis disappeared, which would suggest that the activity of the left hemisphere in maintaining an hysterical paralysis had been inhibited.

This hemiplegic state lasted some three months; then, following a slight hysterical attack, he awoke the following morning back to normal with no recollection of his hemiplegic state and in a noisy, quarrelsome state reminiscent of his thieving days at Bonneval.

He escaped from Bicêtre after stealing money and clothes but was soon arrested and convicted, and was sent to Rochefort Asylum, where he promptly threw an hysterical fit which returned him into a state of hysterical right hemiplegia.

In Rochefort Drs Bourru and Burot experimented on Louis V with a variety of treatments popular at that time, which, in my opinion, were just another form of strong suggestion. We know from Dr Voisin that Louis V was a very good hypnotic subject and easily hypnotized.

From their experiments Drs Bourru and Burot were able to recognize no fewer than six different personalities and, to quote directly from Dr Myers's paper:

> [They] . . . lay great stress on their observations that not only are these past and forgotten mental states recalled by physical impressions, but also conversely, if a past and forgotten mental state is suggested to the patient as his actual and present condition he accepts this belief, and with it comes back his past physical condition.
>
> For example if Louis V was told positively and authoritatively that he was in Bonneval in March, 1880, with Dr Camuset, he would not only lose memory both of his subsequent and early life, and take up the boyish manners and tailor's habits of that period, but would also show the paraplegia and contracture of the legs, and anaesthesia of the lower part of the body; and in the same way other suggestions of time and place and mental state brought with them their historically appropriate physical accompaniments.

This I would expect if the patient were in hypnosis.

Dr Myers goes on to say:

> [Drs Bourru and Burot] . . . do not feel Dr Voisin's or indeed any theory of double personality sufficient to cover the facts of the case as they have shown them; they consider it as a case of Multiple Personality, but they regard any exact interpretation as at present hazardous. They are inclined, however, to believe in a dual action of the brain, and in the probably unstable

predominance of either hemisphere in a case such as this. They point to the imperfect speech and violent character associated with the right hemisphere at Bicêtre and Rochefort, in contrast to the clear speech and self-controlled manners at Saint Urbain etc., as showing the different tendencies of the supremacy of the left and right hemispheres.

We leave the nineteenth century with the phenomenon of dual (or multiple) personality becoming more recognized by the medical profession, along with the realization that hypnosis held the key to exposure of the personalities and had a role to play in its therapy.

Unfortunately, this interest was not to continue. The early part of the twentieth century was denuded of research into this intriguing human behaviour by what I can only descibe as the 'Freudian hypnotic gap'. During the first quarter of this century the use of hypnosis was largely ignored or even ridiculed by the medical profession in favour of the growing popularity of movements based on psychoanalytic theory.

Such terms as 'Freudian', 'Jungian' or 'Adlerian' were household words and had an unparalleled influence on the development of twentieth-century psychological and psychiatric thought. It was not until the neurological investigations of Roger Sperry exploded into the world of human mental processes that interest in the possibility of a dual mind revived. The diagnosis of multiple personality once more became a subject to research, and in 1985 the *American Diagnostic and Statistical Manual of Mental Disorders* acknowledged its existence and gave it a definition.

The latest publication of this manual (*DSM 3R*, 1987) states this to be:

A) The existence within the person of two or more distinct personalities or personality states (each with its own enduring pattern of perceiving, relating to, and thinking about the environment and self).
B) At least two of these personality states recurrently take full control of the person's behaviour.

It was the keen interest shown in the 1980s by American psychologists and psychiatrists that led to its recognition. Of these, particular mention should be made of the work of R.P. Kluft, who has published several papers on the multiple personality syndrome, and Professor Eugene L. Bliss of the University of Utah whose book *Multiple Personality, Allied Disorders and Hypnotism* (1986) shows intriguing insight and originality.

From my personal point of view the possibility of multiple personalities occurring in human beings was always a valid theoretical concept. After all, an adult human being has been shown by Roger Sperry to be made up of two distinct individuals, each of whom, under circumstances entailing a loss of inter-connecting pathways, acts independently of the other. Is there any evidence to support that this can occur in individuals with a normal brain structure?

Peggy Gott, Everett Hughes and Katherine Whipple (1984)[5] gave a case history of a thirty-one-year-old, right-handed woman who had the ability to switch voluntarily and quickly between two different and emotional patterns or personalities. Her two personalities she called 'me' and 'it'. 'Me' was essentially a logical, mathematical, organized businesswoman who was easily angered at inefficiency – typical left hemisphere characteristics. 'It', in contrast, enjoyed sports like tennis, was relaxed and sexy – typical of right hemisphere characteristics. Electroencephalograms taken in her 'me' phase confirmed more left than right hemisphere activity and similarly more right than left hemisphere activity when functioning as 'it'. Further confirmation of this shift in cerebral dominance was obtained by measuring the time taken for stimuli to cross from one hemisphere to the other (interhemispheric transmission time). The experimenters concluded that this woman could work on either her left or right hemisphere at will.

This case appears to support the Sperry concept that 'we are *two* beings in one bony cranium', and yet clinically, it is often possible to identify three or four or more personalities. Is it possible to explain these in similar neurological terms?

Obviously, any thoughts on this subject must be speculative, but my experience with the hypnotic phenomenon has led me to believe *that the presence of multiple personalities is a normal characteristic of human beings and that they are the result of normal learning processes which in themselves are part of a mental defence mechanism.*

Let me further explain this conjecture.

'Which hat are you wearing now?' is a well-known, everyday expression, which uses the word 'hat' as a synonym for a character or personality not usually recognized as the norm for the specific individual in question.

All of us, from time to time, wear different hats, and in my opinion, with each hat goes a personality.

The soccer fan with brightly coloured shirt, tasselled cap and a 6-foot-long scarf, swaying and singing on 'the kop' before the match, hurling insults at rival fans during the match, reeling from pub to pub after the match, cannot possibly be the same individual who that morning, as an undertaker's assistant, walked slowly and solemnly behind the hearse, wearing sub-fusc and with topper lowered in reverence.

The totally intolerant ENT surgeon, green-gowned and gloved, pacing up and down the side of the operating table snorting at the inefficiency of the theatre staff through his impatient mask. The pale-faced house-surgeon waiting his turn to catch the wrongly selected instruments as they are hurled back at the hand that proffered them. This bellowing, bombastic senior surgeon could not possibly be the same man who, that afternoon, laughingly apologized to his partner as he missed a 2-foot putt on the sixteenth green to lose the match, then shook hands warmly with his opponents saying how he had enjoyed the game. One of them, the house-surgeon, could not believe it was the same man.

In both these cases, as in the case published by Gott, two distinct modes of behaviour are all too apparent, but they are occurring in people whom all of us would consider *normal and well-orientated*.

It is easy to pick out which hemisphere is dominant. Always the left hemisphere is the 'logical controller', inhibiting any behaviour unseemly to the occasion and, as such, fulfilling a protective role for the individual.

The young undertaker's assistant, solemnly carrying out his duties, would soon lose his job if his behaviour were not firmly under the control of his logical hemisphere. That is not to say that his thoughts as he followed the cortège were not on the afternoon's match!

The surgeon, although seemingly intolerant and liable to flare up, nevertheless is working on his left hemisphere. He is maintaining the logical precision of the responsible surgeon with a life in his hands, and to do this he must pounce on any slackness or errors in his staff that could jeopardize this responsibility. He may be well aware of the anxiety and discomfort his behaviour generates among his staff, but working on his left hemisphere this is not interpreted in an emotionally sympathetic way but with a cold, logical disdain for their incompetence and a logical desire to make them sit up and learn!

To follow further this line of reasoning. Perhaps one of the most perplexing instances of human behaviour was that of the staff of the German concentration camps (such as Buchenwald) during the Second World War. How could so-called 'normal' inhabitants of villages surrounding these camps possibly take on a job in these camps knowing full well the nature of the horrors being perpetrated inside their gates? How could, say, a married German villager tolerate the sight of those living and dead skeletons, then go home to his family and children at the end of the day as a normal loving father?

Surely the daytime worker and the nighttime father are two completely incompatible individuals.

These questions have haunted present-day psychiatrists, psychologists and philosophers, simply because the natural answer would be *to condemn these camp workers outright as mentally deranged.* But, except for a very few extremists, all the evidence points to the majority of the German concentration-camp employees falling within a *normal mental category.*

It seems to me that a possible explanation could lie in the ability of these workers to separate their personalities. If this is so, then it would appear that their left logical hemisphere had been persuaded, or manipulated, into believing that a certain belief or behaviour was logically correct. Once this is established in the mind of the individual, then it appears possible to carry out any form of atrocity under the cloak of its being 'justifiable'. These workers' daytime personalities logically identified the camp inmates as enemies so dangerous that they must be destroyed, and as they were functioning on a logical and non-emotional hemisphere, this personality did not turn a hair at the sight of such suffering.

History is full of instances of such inexplicable behaviour.

The social record, for instance, of religious fundamentalist belief (whatever denomination one cares to name) is simply appalling! The slave trade, the Inquisition and the fatwahs are typical examples. One could argue that fundamentalism only flourishes in backward communities where education is at a minimum and survival often depends on primitive moral codes of behaviour which would be condemned in a more sophisticated environment. This is an attractive argument in so far as it would explain the ease with which atrocities such as genocide can occur under such conditions, and also how the lack of moral education leaves the logical hemisphere vulnerable to manipulation in order to justify such deeds. I am sure this view may indeed be correct in explaining many of the Third World's atrocities, but it is certainly not the only explanation.

In 1964, the Socio-psychological Prize of the American Association for the Advancement of Science was awarded to Stanley Milgram for his work *Obedience to Authority*.[6,7] He took a large number of volunteers (both male and female) from all ages and occupations, and told them he was conducting an experiment to establish the effect of punishment on learning. They, the volunteers, were to be the teachers, and they were to administer an electric shock to pupils whenever they gave a wrong answer to a question (the pupils were wired to an electric chair in a separate room). The strength of the electric shock was to increase with each successive wrong answer up to a point where it was possible actually to kill the pupil!

The pupils were, in fact, actors and no shocks were ever given, but the teachers were completely unaware of this. The actors screamed with pain and pleaded with the experimenter to stop the shocks, but he refused and demanded that the teacher continue.

Milgram's results were astounding and very disturbing. They showed that it was possible to persuade 62 per cent of the volunteers to press the button which would have effectively *killed* the pupil! As one might expect, this experiment has caused endless discussion in moral circles, all of which have given a variety of cogent reasons to explain how apparently normal individuals within a Western environment can stoop to such extraordinary behaviour.

In my opinion there is one more possible explanation; this can lie in the human ability to become another personality.

As under the Nazi hegemony, the experimenter has induced, by false logic and authoritative bullying, a very powerful conflict in an individual (the teacher) who would not normally carry out such an immoral act. A conflict of such a powerful nature threatens the very survival of the teacher's personality, and the teacher has to call up an extreme defence mechanism to prevent a mental breakdown.

As I have previously suggested, the result could be the development of another, separate personality who has the logical reasoning and emotional inhibition to kill.

A sinister hat to add to their rack!

I have tried to show that we can recognize multiple personality behaviour in so-called normal individuals. If this is so, then multiple personality must be considered as a normal human characteristic.

I have also put forward the hypothesis that the production of multiple personalities is part of human learning processes, processes which in themselves are part of the mental defence mechanism.

What is left to consider are those individuals who *suffer* as a result of multiple personalities; that is, patients who are diagnosed as suffering from a multiple personality *disorder*, and whether hypnosis can be of help in these cases. In order to do this I think we should take a more detailed look at fantasy.

All of us, at whatever age, possess the ability to fantasize, some of us to a much greater extent than others, and some to such an extreme degree that their fantasies sometimes take on flesh, as it were, and become apparitions. The identification of the existence of individuals with this capability I consider important in explaining the origin and mechanism of multiple personality disorder, as well as the use of hypnosis in its treatment.

Let us take the case history of a child who, at the age of ten, was raped by her father. Shall we say that up to this incident the child's life had been relatively happy and her relationship with her parents of a loving intimacy one would normally expect within a family. The child had friends with whom she played, and more often than not their games involved fantasy, such as 'doctors and nurses' or 'mummies and daddies' or 'school' and so on.

Occasionally, if the child were by herself, she would conjure up an imaginary playmate or give varying characters to her dolls, which she would scold or praise according to the imaginary behaviour she endowed to each one. For instance, 'Mary was a good doll because she ate up all her vegetables' but 'Joan was very bad because she threw her plate on the floor!' Soon the personalities of Mary and Joan would become more and more complex, but always it was Joan who was the bad character. In her play the child was introjecting the moral code of her environment, and 'Mary', who knew the correct, logical way to behave, became her moral ideal, whereas 'Joan' was emotionally uncontrollable and bad.

The father then began to take a sexual interest in his daughter, which eventually led up to his total loss of control. During this period it would have been possible to observe a change come over the child's fantasy play-pattern, and the Joan doll's misdemeanours would take on sexual overtones.

The shock of the rape would almost certainly be unexpected, rather like a sudden horrific crash of the school bus, normally a vehicle in which she would have felt very safe. Her immediate mental reaction would be one of terror and *bewilderment*: 'My father would never do this to me', 'Why should he do this to me?', 'What have I done?', and then 'Is it my fault?' The possibility of guilt would prevent her 'admitting' the rape, and gradually another pattern of mental defence in which the whole incident would take the shape of a terrible fantasy would develop, where 'Joan' was both the victim and the culprit.

It did not happen to 'me', it happened to 'it'. Or, *It was not 'me' who did it, it was 'it'.*

One of the problems of this method of defence is that it involves the distortion of memory not only in identification but also in *time*. If the rape was the only one that occurred, in all probability the incident would be frozen to the time period in which it happened and repressed in memory as an unwelcome fantasy, just as it is often impossible to remember the details of a bad dream. On the other hand, as so often happens, the sexual abuse (or even the possibility of it) continues, then the time period becomes of such a length that it is impossible to dismiss this behaviour as a memory of a fantasy.

In order to accommodate this reality, a second personality who indulges in this behaviour becomes itself a reality. But this second personality is not tolerable and must be repressed at all costs.

Such is the strength of the repression that it may become unconscious and therefore unknown to the normal personality, only to surface on certain occasions (probably as the result of some trigger factor), when it is seen to take over full control of the person's behaviour.

We know that children have a great capacity for fantasy. We also know that it is in childhood, when fantasy plays a major role in human learning processes, that these 'other' personalities first appear.

Dr Eugene Bliss has reported a study of fourteen patients with multiple personality disorder, all of whom first developed their other personalities in childhood to help them cope with some traumatic event.

It would appear that the capability of fantasizing plays an important part in the formation of multiple personalities, and it would follow that individuals who are very adept at fantasizing are more likely to suffer from them.

We know that children are extremely good hypnotic subjects. We also know that, under hypnosis, an individual can conjure up a fantasy to such an extent that they firmly believe the room in which they are standing is empty, whereas in truth it is filled with an audience. In other words, a person in a state of hypnosis is so extremely adept at fantasizing that it is often possible to suggest to this hypnotized individual that the (real) person sitting next to them on their right is also sitting next to them on their left! I have often demonstrated this example of an apparition to medical audiences.

But we know of people, who without recourse to hypnosis, experience apparitions of such a nature that their reality seems never in doubt. One such example is the woman patient described by Dr Morton Schatzman in his book *The Story of Ruth* (1980).[8]

Under laboratory investigations it was shown that this patient's apparitions were so real that when she was asked to interpose an apparition of her daughter between herself and a light source in the shape of a standard lamp, her brain actually blotted out the light from this lamp! This patient was also a very good hypnotic subject.

Dr Theodore Xenophon Barber, an American psychologist working in a hospital in Massachusetts and investigating somnambules (individuals extremely susceptible to hypnotic instruction), found to his surprise that out of thirty women somnambules all could perform hypnotic-type feats *without* the recourse to hypnosis. He states:

> These people did not need to be hypnotised at all. They could summon apparitions, feel heat or cold to order, experience amnesia or blindness, completely of their own free will . . .
> These women had hallucinations and fantasies that were so life-like that they tended to confuse memories of fantasies with memories of reality. The amazing thing is that most were

ordinary women living normal lives and unaware that they could do, and experience, things other people could not!

All the women had fantasized from childhood and continued to fantasize as adults. These women were not patients and did not complain of any psychological problems.

It is well known to doctors practising hypnotherapy that the psychoneurotic patient tends to be a good hypnotic subject. Dr Bliss, in his studies of multiple personality disorder,[9] has come to believe that, in this condition, the patient hypnotizes himself or herself; he takes the view that the condition *is a form of self-hypnosis*. In a similar vein, an American professor, Martin Orne, has found phobic patients to be highly hypnotizable; the more suggestible they were, the more phobias they suffered. He has concluded that phobics frequently fall into hypnotic states in which they confuse reality and fantasy and in doing so create their irrational fears.

In conclusion, the condition of multiple personality confirms the human ability to possess at least two personalities, which can be so different as to be at loggerheads with each other.

There is ample evidence, in my opinion, that multiple personality possession does not constitute an abnormal mental state in so far as it can be observed in apparently normal individuals. Where multiple personalities show as a serious mental illness their origin can, almost without exception, be traced back to traumatic events in their childhood, and evidence would suggest that their formation was a method by which they attempted to cope.

Hypnosis, in its ability not only to expose the presence of these personalities but also to make communication with them possible, must be considered an essential part of any therapy designed to help solve any mental disorder associated with them. Cameral analysis is one such therapy.

Chapter 10

The case history of Mrs Susan X

AUTHOR'S NOTE ON THE CASE HISTORY OF MRS SUSAN X

For reasons which will become very obvious to the reader, the case history of Mrs Susan X has been written so as to preserve the anonymity of all the individuals portrayed. Facts relating to Susan X's emotional life have been fully preserved, but names, places and sometimes occupations have been disguised out of recognition.

The two points that favoured my choice of this patient's history are, first, that I consider her problem to be essentially a 'pure' case. By 'pure' I mean that it occurred in an apparently stable individual who suffered a very unexpected *unconscious* shock which in effect meant a complete negation of her main emotional ambitions in life. I have little doubt in my mind that had this woman been spared her unconscious shock she would have coped with all life's vagaries in a competent manner without ever suffering from panic attacks.

On the other hand, I have many similar cases about whom I would have considerable doubts. For instance, one of my patients developed panic attacks at the age of twenty-five which usually came on when she was travelling in public transport (train or bus). This patient's past history was horrifying. Her father came home drunk every Friday night (pay-day was Friday) and proceeded to beat up his wife. My patient remembers her mother hiding behind her for protection when she was only five years old. She ran away from home at the age of fourteen. She was made a 'ward of court' and eventually put in the care of her uncle (her mother's brother), who then sexually abused her.

The number of onion-skins I had to peel off this individual to expose her problems were never-ending, and some may still remain. The problem with giving this type of case history is that its complexity could cause confusion and interpretations could justifiably vary.

Which brings me to the second reason for the choice of Susan X. Analytical treatment of anxiety states, of which panic attacks and phobias are examples, often involves hard work on the part of the analyst in uncovering significant incidents in the patient's past history. The extent to which the analyst has to probe and the minutiae of detail to be exposed often determine a successful outcome. At the risk of boring the reader with its length, I decided on the case of Susan X because I think it best illustrates this point. At the same time it demonstrates the methodology of cameral analysis and emphasizes the asymmetrical nature of knowledge in what I hope to be a fairly simple and understandable way.

'JUST A TYPICAL NORFOLK HOUSEWIFE'

Mrs X was aged twenty-eight when she first consulted me and her doctor's letter of referral read as follows:

Dear Dr Pedersen

Re: Mrs. X d.o.b. 30/7/42
(address)

This patient, whom I have known for many years, suddenly developed what I can only describe as panic attacks, and, at the same time, her sleep pattern became disturbed.

The first symptoms occurred about two months ago when she was watching an innocuous current affairs programme on the television with her husband.

Evidently she turned to her husband, gripped his hand and said that she felt very frightened but had no idea why. The attack passed off after about five minutes and she thought no more about it until a week later when the same feeling came over her whilst she was rolling out the pastry for some mince-pies she was making. Like the first one, the attack came quite out of the blue and for apparently no reason, but this time she came out in a cold sweat and her hands began to tremble.

The attacks are now more frequent, sometimes occurring twice in a day, they all follow the same pattern and when they pass off she feels fine, there is no obvious trigger factor and they occur at any time of the day or night.

Obviously with this history she had to be fully investigated and the results of the tests are enclosed. As you can see they are all within normal limits.

The reluctant conclusion is that her symptoms are hysterical in origin, a view supported by the psychiatrist to whom she was referred and who has recommended a course of tranquillizers.

This, however, has created a problem. Mrs. X came off the pill about five months ago. Her first child is now just over two years old and both she and her husband are anxious to get on with creating their family (I believe Mrs. X is keen on having three or even four children) but she refuses to take any drugs whilst there is a possibility of her becoming pregnant.

I must say, after thalidomide, her attitude is very understandable, hence my referring her to you to see if hypnotherapy can help.

This case puzzles me. The family is well-to-do and very well liked in the area. They are fairly regular church-goers and have always appeared to me to be very sensible, well-adjusted individuals who call a spade a spade. I am surprised to see Mrs. X in the role of an hysteric – it just does not fit!

To me Mrs. X has always been just a typical Norfolk housewife who gives the impression of being able to cope with any of life's difficulties, but I would be grateful for your opinion.

Yours sincerely,

The sheaf of photostat copies of all the examinations and investigations carried out, both by her doctor and the consultants at the hospital she attended, accompanied the letter. They clearly eliminated any physical or organic cause for her symptoms and added up to a robust picture of good health.

Many times in my life patients have been referred to me complaining of symptoms which at first sight appear to be purely psychological in origin. Nevertheless, in the course of taking their history, or perhaps following a further investigation, and sometimes as a result of their mode of response to my form of treatment, another diagnosis emerges pointing to a physical origin. Mrs X, at this stage, does not appear to fall into this category of patient, although her doctor cannot quite accept the neurotic label and takes pains to point out the down-to-earth normality of the whole family. He then emphasizes this stability by a subtle ethnic observation that implies that typical Norfolk house-wives can cope with life very well and are not usually subject to nervous complaints. These two points are very interesting because what has puzzled the doctor actually tells us where conflicts are liable to occur, conflicts that could be the origin of the panic attacks.

If, as her doctor states, the family is well-to-do and very well liked in the area, then its members must be recognized as having set themselves a very high moral standard. We have a fairly accurate idea of this standard because we are told that the family are regular church (of England?) attenders.

Should any member transgress this moral code, then he or she knows that not only have they let *themselves* down but also the whole family, which could greatly enhance the guilt. Here, then, is a possible source of inner conflict which could engender anxiety.

What is also interesting is the suggestion by the doctor that regional characteristics may be used to predict a pattern of behaviour.

Mrs X has the reputation of being, at least in her doctor's experienced eyes, precisely that typical Norfolk housewife who should be strong enough to cope with any of life's difficulties, and I have no doubt that her friends in that category probably see her in the same way. One of the expected ways of behaviour of this group, as implied by her doctor, is to exhibit a high degree of mental stability.

If Mrs X were to fail in this she would react with shame at the thought of letting down her immediate environmental principles, absorbed into her character from childhood, and which point her out as a Norfolk housewife rather than someone from, say, an inner-city, drug-orientated environment. It could be argued that underlying the left hemisphere's logical decision to refuse the drug treatment proferred by the psychiatrist may be the right hemi-sphere's emotional reasoning that 'being under a psychiatrist' becomes a derisive remark when uttered by a typical Norfolk housewife! Here we have another possible source of anxiety, which could, by its very environmental strength, overwhelm that phlegmatic approach of the traditional Norfolk housewife and give rise to her symptoms.

It is possible then, from the doctor's letter, tentatively to determine certain lines of approach to the patient's problem, but until the all-important first interview they must remain only tentative. Very often the impression gained from medical reports, whatever their source, has too great an influence on subsequent investigation and may actually delay progress by compounding an error of judgement. This is particularly true where the problem is psychological in origin. One colleague of mine even goes so far as to refuse to read reports from his psychiatric social workers until *after* his first interview with the patient. This is not because he has lost faith in his assistants; on the contrary, it is because he feels that in this way he gets yet another, totally unbiased, impression from which to work.

The first interview with any patient is all-important. It is not only where the patient's confidence in the therapy must be initiated but also, from the doctor's point of view, where an adequate insight into the patient's psychological make-up must be established in order to formulate future treatment patterns. None of this can be achieved in 5 minutes. The length of the first interview is not determined by the time-allowance of the appointment.

More often than not, two, or even on occasions three sessions may be necessary before any form of active therapy can be started although, of course, a certain amount of passive therapy begins as soon as the patient walks through the door!

All medical students are taught in their clinical years a routine method of taking a patient's case history which is designed to reveal as much information as possible relevant to the presenting symptoms. By making this a routine procedure it is unlikely that any significant elements will be overlooked that could be vital in formulating a diagnosis.

With the patient in front of him, and prior to the physical examination, the doctor goes through a verbal routine of questions concerning the history of the presenting condition (HPC), the patient's past history (PH), family history (FH) and so on, writing notes on the answers he receives. The doctor then follows this up with another set of routine questions specific to the various systems of the body, such as the central nervous system (CNS), the respiratory system (RS), the cardio-vascular system (CVS) and so forth, until a detailed medical picture of the patient's problem is revealed.

Armed with this verbal information, the ensuing physical examination can be conducted with more precision and this in turn will lead to a more accurate diagnosis.

This is a tried and tested method. It works perfectly well for the majority of physical ailments and is, indeed, all that is necessary for the correct diagnosis and treatment of the patient.

It stands to reason, however, that where the problem is psychogenic in origin a much more sophisticated interview is necessary.

To the good, routine medical history outlined above must be added a psychiatric history, which includes questions on inter-personal relationships both at home and work, childhood experiences, social factors, ambitions, and any other aspects of life that may have contributed to the patient's psychological make-up. Then again, the patient's mode of conversation is all-important. Does he react quickly or sluggishly, does he find it difficult to formulate words, are his answers bizarre or logical, has he areas of amnesia, is his perception normal or has he experienced illusions, delusions, hallucinations? Furthermore, a psychiatrist will make notes of any agitation or depression, the degree of awareness and orientation the patient has towards his surroundings both in time and place, his mood and general emotional behaviour.

The value of interpreting the patient's body-language during an interview is well recognized and the majority of psychiatrists make good use of it, noting in particular such things as appearance, gestures and body attitudes. To me, however, it has a greatly added importance in so far as it is the 'language' of the right hemisphere and as such is one of the techniques of cameral analysis used to interpret the views and emotions of that hemisphere.

My 'first' interview with Mrs X took up two appointments, and from it I was able to draw up this picture of this 'typical Norfolk housewife'.

She entered the room slowly with a slight air of suspicion as if feeling her way, but as I rose from my chair and came round from the desk to greet her, she smiled, and the slightly suspicious look gave way to a look of more tolerable acceptance as she lifted her hand to shake mine. She had thin, long fingers and a firm grasp.

Mrs X was undoubtedly a very good-looking woman. She was a bit above average in height, had shoulder-length dark brown hair and pale blue eyes. Her perfect feminine figure had a suppleness which, combined with her long legs, gave a distinct sensual appearance to her movements as she crossed the room to the chair I had offered her in front of the desk.

Mrs X was wearing a dark, two-piece suit made of a thin material and well-fitting. Under the jacket she wore a cream-coloured silk blouse unbuttoned at the neck but sporting a yellow and black spotted silk cravat held in position by a gold clip in the shape of a riding-crop. Her stockings toned in with her skirt and her black shoes were sensible London walking brogues, light-weight but smart. I noticed a small gold watch on her left wrist and a heavy gold ornamental bangle on the right. The colour scheme, although dark grey, was not drab, and the bright offset of yellow and gold produced an impression of smart efficiency which totally denied any depressive interpretation. The just noticeable scent she used was distinct but subtle and male-attractive.

The whole picture added up to an elegant, well-dressed woman, slightly expensive but at the same time discreet, sensible, and what is more, obviously in command of herself.

The only sign of any underlying anxiety was the posture she assumed as she positioned herself in the chair. She sat a shade towards the edge, leaning slightly forward with her legs crossed and her hands in her lap.

It was a defensive position. She was on guard.

I opened up with the usual disparaging remark about the weather; it had no meaning but came over as a kindly noise and established an 'Englishness' which offered no threat.

Very slowly, as the interview progressed, Mrs X relaxed and her answers became less stereotyped and more character-informative; less verbal, more holistic; less guarded, more useful. As her history unfolded she increasingly clothed the bare words with a slightly more emotional dressing; a light laugh or a cynical obser-vation, a poignant gesture or a meaningful look, a witty remark or a condemning explanation. Gradually, as her tight verbal cage loosened up, she allowed more emotive words to slip out, and always, waiting to surround them like some excited reception party, were body-signals anxious to emphasize their agreement and rejoicing in their freedom to be expressed. A remembered caress with an accompanied blush, a crude expletive with an angry flush, a melancholy tear.

Eventually Mrs X was able fully to communicate.

There was nothing she felt she needed to hide or hold back from me. Nothing was going to upset me, nothing was going to shock me. She felt totally free to express, in any way whatsoever, whatever she felt like expressing, knowing that this was necessary for the understanding of her problem. She knew that she was safe and under no threat, no risk of exposure, no hint of ridicule and no possibility of punishment.

When this stage is reached progress is rapid.

This is the stage where the patient's mental roles are reversed.

The emotional hemisphere is at last given its head and appears to have persuaded the verbal hemisphere to relinquish its dominant and censorial role and instead take on the totally passive job of helping to interpret emotional viewpoints in terms of verbal language.

This is poetry without the syntactical rules and is therapeutic in its own right.

It is the closest point one can reach to the understanding of purely emotional motives without altering the state of consciousness. To progress further one needs to eliminate the verbal hemisphere altogether and to open up the involuntary memory store (specific to the emotional hemisphere) and let the patient rediscover the origins of the problem. This will come later; in the meanwhile, here is her history up to the onset of her problem as I recorded it from her verbal statements.

Stage one of cameral analysis

Mrs X was an only child. She was extremely fond of her parents and got on with them well. She knew her parents would do anything for her but denied that she had been 'spoilt'; in fact, at times she felt that they had almost gone out of their way to avoid such an accusation, particularly in her adolescent years and with the growth of their affluence. Her father we will call Jack A.

Jack A left school in 1934 at the age of sixteen to become a clerk in a coal-merchant's office. His boss was a bachelor friend of his father, and it was generally assumed that if the lad showed promise and was up to the job, he would be eventually offered a partnership with the object of taking over the business. It was a good business and the prospects were also good.

Jack had joined the Territorial Army in 1938 and, as a result, was called up immediately war was declared in 1939. He opted for Army transport and maintains he owes his life and his post-war success to that decision. Being in transport, he was able to make the Dunkirk beaches without much difficulty and survived the sea evacuation.

While on leave in 1941 he married a girl he had known since she was fourteen, and their daughter, my patient Mrs X, was born in 1942.

Within six months of marriage, Jack A was posted to the Middle East as a transport sergeant in the Eighth Army and subsequently saw service in Italy and finally in North Germany.

When he was demobbed in 1946 he was a totally different individual from the one who had occupied the clerk's desk in the station-yard office of the coal-merchant. He no longer wished to be anything other than his own boss. He had, as he put it, survived not only the enemy but the Army itself, the latter, in his opinion, being the greater achievement! Jack was, furthermore, well versed in the transport business and realized the importance of oil.

He declined the offer of taking up his old job but remained on good terms with his pre-war employer and actually rented part of the station yard from him.

He bought an Army surplus road haulage tanker for a knock-down price and went into the fuel-oil business. Within eighteen months he had six Army surplus tankers and three men working for him and contracts to supply heating oils to a local Army and Air Force base in the vicinity. By 1960 he owned a fleet of tankers and two filling-stations; he bought out the coal-merchant purely for the convenience of the station-yard premises, and they lived in the farmhouse of the very farm on which his wife had worked. He was worth a bob or two!

Mrs X's mother, Mrs Mary A, was also an only child. Her father was a Methodist minister and the family moved around the country at regular intervals.

She met her future husband, Jack A, at a dance in the Methodist hall.

Mary was a physically mature fourteen-year-old but innocent and extrovert. She persuaded a reluctant Jack A onto the dance floor and soon had his adolescent shyness lost in a welter of new emotions. She reflected another image of himself, which he found flattering and they both enjoyed exploring each other's company.

Jack was four years older and Mary was still at school; neverthe-less they looked a good pair, obviously happy together, and they became inseparable. The innocence and openness of their re-lationship was accepted by both sets of parents and as the years progressed their eventual marriage was looked upon as a natural outcome whenever it became economically viable.

The advent of war blasted Jack and Mary's world to uncertainty. The future was no longer possible to predict. Recognized patterns of behaviour became obsolete and 'one crowded hour of glorious life' became an acceptable theme for young warriors. Dunkirk settled the matter.

Despite her age (she was under twenty-one) Mary received her parent's permission to marry Jack and her father performed the ceremony on a wet Friday afternoon in 1941. The reception was held in the same hall in which they had met, and their honeymoon was spent in a country-house hotel some 10 miles away. Jack returned to his unit on the Sunday evening. One of their wedding presents was a good-luck sack of coal, a small piece of which Jack carried around with him throughout the war. It is now mounted on a little square of white marble and sits on his desk at home.

The newly-weds met sporadically over the next six months whenever Jack could scrounge a pass. Sometimes he was able to get home, but mainly those brief hours together were spent walking, if the weather was fine, or in a cinema or tea-room, if inclement. Occasionally, they were able to spend the night together in some boarding-house near the barracks.

Jack was posted to the Middle East in early 1942 and did not see his wife or his child (born later that year) until December 1944, when his unit was transferred from Italy to Germany. He was granted three weeks' leave while his unit was refitted in England.

Just after she married and before she became pregnant, Mary started work as a Land Girl on a 1,000-acre farm owned by a friend of her father. It was an ideal arrangement. Not only was she able to live at home (the farm was less than a mile away) but the Land Army was a reserved occupation and exempted her from any call-up to the women's services. So throughout this period of separation from her husband and the birth of their daughter, Mary lived at home with her parents and continued to help on the farm whenever she could.

Apart from the obvious anxiety about the welfare of her husband, it was a stable and happy time for the family and an ideal environment for the baby.

Mrs X was born Susan M.A., and weighed 7 pounds 4 ounces. Her mother's pregnancy had been uneventful, and the labour, although somewhat prolonged in the early stages, was otherwise normal. Susan was born at home and delivered by the local midwife. She was breast-fed up to the age of fourteen months and weaned without incident. She was a very happy child, sat up at six months and walked well at one year. Her appetite was good, and apart from the odd times she cut a tooth, slept throughout the night and there was no doubt that she was a great joy to her mother and grandparents.

Susan first saw her father when she was two-and-a-half years old.

It was Christmas 1944. Jack had returned with his unit from Italy and was on leave prior to their joining Montgomery's section of the Rhine Army.

Naturally, this was an intensely emotional moment for the family and is well remembered by them all. Furthermore, the whole period was permanently recorded by Jack using an expensive German camera he had 'acquired' in Italy especially for such a purpose. Remembered by all, that is, except Susan, whose memory of this event is purely from being shown, in later years, the excellent photographs her father had taken at the time with his 'new' Leica.

The first memories of her childhood Susan can consciously recall are those associated with their move from her grandparents' house. She was four at the time, and clearly remembers both her mother and father helping her to pack up all her toys into a big wicker basket, which they then loaded very carefully into a large van. Their new house was semi-detached and situated in a cul-de-sac on the other side of the town. After nearly six years of marriage it was the first home of their own and a much looked-forward-to occasion.

In the two years they spent in this house Jack laid the foundations of his fuel-oil business and his wife was the unpaid secretary. They both worked extremely hard and never took a holiday. What spare time they had they spent with their child. Mary took Susan to a kindergarten school in the morning and her grandparents collected her after lunch, and in doing so maintained to a large extent the continuity of life the child had previously enjoyed. What might have been a traumatic wrench followed by a period of parental neglect turned out to be as smooth a transition as possible under the circumstances, and in no way was Susan exposed to any significant stress. By the time they came to move again two years later, Susan was that much older, had made some nice friends at school, and was well able to cope with yet another new environment.

It is worth mentioning at this point that, on looking back on her life, Susan had no recollection of any period of time when her father was not at home with them. It would appear, then, that another transition, the replacing of grandfather with father, had been expertly handled by the whole family and there was no evidence whatsoever of any associated emotional trauma.

The move to the farm had been a difficult financial decision for Jack to make, particularly as it had had to be made in a hurry. The property had come onto the market as the result of a compulsory purchase order on a section of the land required for a new bypass. This effectively cut the farm in two and lowered its viability as a single profitable unit. The farmhouse with 150 acres was left on one side of the road and the remaining 840 was on the other. Mary, you remember, had been a Land Girl on this farm for part of the war, and had always known of the existence of this compulsory purchase order, which had been lodged on the land since 1937 but which had been effectively put on ice by that war.

Because of her close association and her father's friendship with the farmer, Mary was probably the first to know that the county was about to take up the purchase order. This gave Jack a few weeks' start on other potential buyers.

The farmhouse, farm buildings, storage sheds and stabling, along with the 150 acres, were exactly what Jack needed for his rapidly expanding business. The rest of the land on the other side of the road he knew could be tacked onto an existing farm whose land was adjacent. Jack also knew that the farmer who owned this adjacent farm had two strapping young sons and could easily cope with the extra acres, but, because of an incident involving the siting of a pig-manure silage in 1936, had been a sworn enemy of his neighbour ever since and would in no way do business with him.

In a piece of spectacular entrepreneurial enterprise, Jack negotiated a massive three-month loan, bought the whole farm for less than its agricultural value because of the impending purchase order, then sold (at auction) 840 acres to the farmer with the two sons at what was a record value for agricultural land at that time. He ended up with the farmhouse and 150 acres at a cost that turned out to be less than the price he obtained for the semi-detached! Not content with that he obtained planning permission to run his fuel-oil business from the farmhouse and to build underground fuel storage tanks and a lorry park on a part of the land easily accessible from the road. At a reunion of his old wartime unit held about this time, some of Jack's friends from the Sergeants' Mess were amused to hear of this successful trans-action, but were not surprised.

The acquisition of the farm had an additional spin-off which was to have a very important influence on both Susan and her mother. Mary had always been a keen horsewoman, but the opportunity to indulge in this sport to any serious degree had always eluded her. Now she had her chance, and her husband gave generous encouragement.

Susan became inspired by her mother's enthusiasm and quickly became a competent rider. A paddock was built and practice fences erected. Horses were bought and trained, and later some were bred on the farm. As their fortunes increased, both mother and daughter became more ambitious and they began eventing seriously; soon rosettes began appearing on the stable doors.

And so a pattern of life was gradually developed which was to become an integral part of family existence; their sporting achiev-ments complemented Jack's business successes and their name became well known in the county. From the age of seven, through adolescence to adulthood, Susan's spare time revolved around horses, but her mother was careful to keep the enthusiasm within bounds and at an amateur level. It was a hobby to be enjoyed but not to be taken too seriously.

Susan's schooling began when she was sent to the kindergarten at the age of five. She left there at the age of seven to attend a small private school. She was taught well at this school and, at the age of eleven, easily passed the entrance exam to the County High School for Girls, which boasted a good academic record. She enjoyed the County High and was popular from the start both among the staff and the girls.

Susan was keen on all forms of sport but her riding successes, which were ex-curricula, made her stand out from other girls and earned her a degree of hero-worship which, she says, she exploited unmercifully. Nowadays, on looking back, she becomes embar-rassed at the thought of some of her actions, but on the whole acknowledges the character-building value of those competitive years.

Susan made many friends at school. Those of them who still live in the area she sees regularly. However, the girl who was to become her greatest friend came from outside her area; they both met at a gymkhana. Susan was almost eleven years old and about to take the entrance exam to the County High. Pamela was nearly thirteen and was just about to leave her preparatory boarding-school for a progressive, mixed, public school in the West Country. They were both at an important period of social change in their lives and they were both vulnerable.

Although Pamela was two years older than Susan, they were the same size as each other and they were both pubescent. Because of the age difference Pamela tended to be the more dominant, but each contributed equally to the friendship. Their interest in horses and skills in eventing brought them together and founded their initial friendship, but as the years progressed they became emotionally closer and soon acted as total confidantes to each other.

Pamela had a younger brother. Her parents tended to be aloof towards their children and expected a high standard of self-control and behaviour from them. Pamela and her brother had been packed off to boarding-schools as soon as they were old enough. This Victorian attitude of the parents had been noticed by the headmistress of Pamela's prep-school, who felt it too restrictive; it was she who, surprisingly, persuaded the parents to choose the progressive, mixed, public school for Pamela instead of the more conventional in the hope of correcting the imbalance.

Susan's parents, on the other hand, were warm and openly affectionate, they trusted their daughter and rarely restricted her activities.

Pamela envied Susan's home life and freedom and wished she had such understanding parents, whereas Susan secretly enjoyed the upper-class aura and public school image portrayed by Pamela and tended to copy her. Both girls met in their holidays at the various events they attended and corresponded with each other during the term-time.

Pamela's new boarding-school was an eye-opener to them both. In the beginning, Susan used to read to her parents parts of Pamela's letters, but by the third term this habit had ceased altogether and her parents were given a very expurgated version of the life at a progressive, mixed, boarding-school in the mid-fifties!

In the summer holidays, one year after their first meeting, Susan was invited to stay with Pamela for a week. Pamela's home was a large, rambling mansion, most of the rooms of which were not in use. The household's activities revolved around the breeding, grooming, training and stabling of up to fifteen horses, five of which belonged to the family; the rest had outside owners. There was a permanent staff of five to run the stables.

Susan's bedroom was next to Pamela's. It was the first time Susan had stayed away from home without her parents and she really looked forward to the occasion. On the first night both girls talked and talked long after they went to bed, and it was inevitable that the sexual experiences of the elder girl were discussed at length. It was equally inevitable that on this holiday Susan learnt of the art and delights of masturbation from her more experienced friend.

Mrs X's memories of this period in her life were very happy and exciting. She enjoyed being part of the household and was a welcome guest. Her obvious competence on horseback and her knowledge of stable routine earned her a satisfying recognition and an acceptance into what was normally a very closed society. In addition, she was seen to be beneficial to Pamela, who had few friends and tended to be reserved. The household staff and the parents were pleased to hear girls' laughter and to see them so obviously enjoying themselves. Visits to each other's homes became a regular occurrence in the summer holidays and occasionally for the odd day in winter and spring.

Susan never felt any guilt about her harmless sexual caprices, and never, even as an adult, considered them in any way abnormal. Masturbation became a regular part of her life and was accompanied by heterosexual fantasies of a loving nature and in keeping with her age and development. By the time she was eighteen there was little doubt that Susan had survived the emotional changes of the pubescent and adolescent years without any undue stress. In addition, she had coped with a degree of achievement in sport that could have spawned problems in less stable individuals.

Susan obtained three reasonable 'A' levels, but her last year at school dragged. She felt she had outgrown the County High and was looking forward to coming out into the world, so she left at eighteen to learn the intricacies of her father's expanding and successful business. In the beginning she was given very much a free hand by her father, who designed her 'office' hours to complement her equestrian interests. At the same time he made sure that she realized, as an only child, that it was also in her interest to have the business at her fingertips.

In searching her past up to this point in her life, Mrs X could pinpoint two incidents which she felt were emotionally significant and which had shocked her at the time they occurred. Even so, she felt that, after her initial reaction, she was soon able to see them in terms of life experience, and it would have surprised her if they were found to relate in a causative way to her panic attacks. One was sexual and one was sad.

The first occurred when she was thirteen.

On Tuesdays and Thursdays in the summer months Susan attended a riding academy some 10 miles from her home. She was picked up by her mother from school in the afternoon and was dropped, along with a canvas bag holding her riding habit, at the entrance to the academy. On this particular day it had been raining and the ground was very muddy with pools of water everywhere.

To save her lightweight school shoes Susan took a short cut to the women's locker room through the large barn used for hay storage. Low wooden partitions sectioned the barn, each section containing different foodstuffs or hay. She was about to pass one of these sections when she heard some odd noises and was surprised to see two figures, one lying and one kneeling, in the hay. She recognized them immediately as being two of the stable lads, both about seventeen years old, and employed by the academy, but it was what they were doing that caused her to freeze. They both had their trousers off. The one lying on his back had a stiff penis, which the other was kneeling over and moving up and down in his mouth; at the same time the penis of the kneeling youth was being moved up and down in the mouth of his friend. To be technical they were in the *soixante-neuf* position and indulging in fellatio. Susan was absolutely shocked and felt rooted to the spot; at the same time she could not keep her eyes off the pair. She slowly pulled herself together and decided that on no account must she be seen, so bent down behind the partition but continued to witness this sexual act until its climax. At this point she quietly retraced her steps, crouching as she went, and let herself out through the same door she had entered.

Describing her feelings about this incident some fifteen years after it had occurred made her realize that, despite the lack of any first-hand personal experience, she could hardly be considered naïve on sexual matters.

She interestingly came to the conclusion that the discussions she had had with her friend Pamela had, as it were, prepared her to accept such a sexual confrontation without any damaging trauma. At the same time she felt that her sex education should not have been left to the Pamelas of this world and that in future she would support the subject as a normal part of any school curriculum!

Nevertheless, the incident was a shock.

She was terrified at the time of being discovered by the boys. She remembers thinking that as her heart was thumping so violently it was bound to be heard. She had never seen an erect male penis before, and she can remember to this day every minute detail of the scene from beginning to end.

How, then, did it affect her? It occupied her thoughts for most of the following week and intruded into her attention to normal school routine. She kept the whole incident to herself and, not trusting a letter, decided to wait until she saw Pamela before letting her in on the secret. Gradually the element of shock disappeared and she actually incorporated the scene into her own sexual fantasies. She became intrigued with the thought of oral sex with a male and came to the conclusion that at some future stage in her life, and given the opportunity with a willing partner, she would not be averse to trying it herself!

The other emotional experience that Susan had considered to be significant was sudden, and sad, and occurred when Susan was seventeen. In the relatively small and somewhat elite world of horsewomen, of which she and her mother were a part, most of the participants were well known to one another. Occasionally the acquaintanceship developed into a more firm friendship, and sometimes, as in the case of Pamela, this extended beyond the 'horsy' environment.

Jane was one such friend of both Susan and Pamela, although not to that special degree enjoyed by the latter pair. Like Susan, Jane was an only child, the daughter of an architect employed in the planning office of an adjacent county. She was small and blonde, a complete extrovert, and bursting with energy and enthusiasm for life. One always knew when she was around, her attractive voice bubbled through any conversation and its scatter-brained content, along with her innocent, blue-eyed expression, was a never-ending source of amusement to all who were listening. But perhaps her most attractive feature was her infectious little laugh. It was impossible not to like Jane and she could be the life and soul of any party. Susan very aptly summed her up when she said that Jane could have been a miniature English stand-in for Goldie Hawn.

Jane was a fearless rider and would tackle anything from the horse to the jump. She fell off more times than average but her small stature seemed to help her avoid any serious injury, and bruising was the most she had ever sustained.

Pamela, although at school, was the first to hear of Jane's accident, through her mother's weekly letter. It had been a misty November morning and Jane was exercising a horse. At one point the bridle path was crossed by a minor road, and Jane brought the horse to a halt to make sure the road was clear. Seeing that it was, she pressed her mount forward but its foreleg slipped on the metalled surface and she was thrown to the ground. Unfortunately, her hard hat came off in the process and she landed on her unprotected head in the middle of the road.

She was picked up almost immediately by a passing car and taken, unconscious, to the nearest hospital, from where she was later transferred to the neurological unit of the county hospital.

Jane lay in a coma for two weeks, then gradually regained consciousness.

Pamela's mother, in relating these facts, implored her daughter to make sure that she fastened her riding hat securely under her chin, but, apart from this warning, the rest of the letter consisted merely of the usual family chit-chat.

It was not surprising, then, that Pamela had the impression that, having recovered consciousness, all was now well with Jane; this impression was further reinforced when she telephoned the hospital and was told that Jane was off the danger list and could receive visitors. Armed with this information Pamela telephoned Susan and together they organized a surprise visit for the following weekend to cheer up Jane. When Susan told her parents of her plans they were disturbed to hear of the accident but relieved to know that all was now well and readily supported the visit, falling in with the idea that it would be a nice surprise.

Pamela obtained permission from the headmaster and travelled up by train. Susan also took a train and they both met under the clock at the station. Pamela was carrying an outrageously large woolly panda (a present for Jane), which triggered off an hilarious meeting much to the amusement of some passers-by. In this happy mood they planned their day over a sandwich lunch in the station buffet. They decided, because of the panda, to take a taxi to the hospital, spend an hour visiting Jane, then catch a bus back to the city in time for a film, before catching the train back to Susan's home where Pamela was staying the night.

From the station buffet they stepped straight into a taxi on the rank and were whisked away to the hospital in no time at all. They enquired at reception the way to the ward and, clutching the giant panda, presented themselves to the ward sister's desk.

It was then only 1.45 p.m. and visiting hour was not until 2.30 p.m. The ward sister was still at lunch and the nurse left in charge had only that morning been allocated to the ward and was not acquainted with Jane's case. She at first told them they would have to wait until 2.30 p.m. but, confronted by a very persuasive pair carrying a large panda, she soon relented and directed them to a small side room at the far end of the ward. The stage was set to cheer up Jane.

The curtains were drawn in the room and the girls took a few seconds to adjust to the low light. They saw a figure propped up in the bed, and as their eyes became accustomed to the gloom they both stared with horror at the sight before them.

She had no hair on her head; there was a livid scar in a large circle above her left temporal region. The whole of the right side of her face drooped and the lower eyelid was everted, exposing the red, watery, inner surface of the mucous membrane. The lips on the right side of her mouth were parted, and from the gap a slow sticky flow of saliva slid down like a thin icicle until it broke off in a blob onto the front lapel of a coarse white, but stained, smock. Her right arm hung loosely and uselessly from her shoulder to a point just below the side of the iron bedstead.

But worse was to come.

The sudden entrance of the girls with the panda had disturbed Jane's half-slumber and, slowly, what was in fact a grin of recognition appeared on the left side of her face – the right side remained immobile. To the onlookers the result was a hideous grimace in which the right side of the mouth was dragged across to the left of the mid-line, exposing the teeth and producing a leering, sardonic expression.

Both Susan and Pamela recoiled involuntarily at this sight and their reaction clearly upset Jane, who now tried desperately to speak to them. The noise she emitted was dreadful – a sort of fluffing roar punctuated by a plopping, spitting sound as the left side of her mouth came together in an attempt to form some sort of words. But it was impossible, Jane's speech centre had been damaged: she would never speak again, she could only make incomprehensible noises.

It was this terrible sound coming from Jane that, along with the shock of her appearance, was just too much for Pamela – she turned towards the door as if to flee the room but instead collapsed in a faint on the floor still clutching the panda. Susan, numbed at first by the encounter, slowly realized the awfulness of the situation, burst into tears and grasped Jane's useless arm as it hung there cold and limp. Jane saw this emotional reaction but could not feel the warmth of the contact and she herself started to cry.

Later, a fully recovered Pamela sat with Susan and the ward sister in a sad little group around Jane's bed, drinking tea. Susan helped Jane drink from a cup with a spout. The ward sister's initial anger had soon turned to empathy as she realized the 'surprise' had been well meant and that the visitors were shocked and chastened.

Susan and Pamela left at 3.00 p.m. and caught the first train home.

Jane was given a sedative and went off to sleep.

The panda found its way discretely to the children's ward.

When Mrs Susan X gave me her verbal description of the incident with Jane she was clearly moved at times by the recollection. Her narrative of the scene in the hospital was broken by short periods of silence, and she had to dab her eyes occasionally with her handkerchief.

Was this then the source of Mrs X's panic attacks?

I feel at this point it is necessary to draw attention to the subtle distinction made, when using cameral analysis, between the emotional shrouding of words.

It is, of course, very natural to react *emotionally* to the *verbal* recall of experiences of this nature, but where cameral analysis is concerned it is possible that this emotional aspect indicates a right hemisphere opinion on the left hemisphere's verbal picture, particularly if it is accompanied by a strong element of body-language.

This possibility should be noted at the point, and whenever it occurs. Let me explain.

The basic principle of cameral analysis, as I have previously intimated, is to compare the verbal hemisphere's interpretation of the patient's problem with that of the non-verbal, emotional hemisphere in order to expose any conflict or discrepancy.

The analysis of the verbal hemisphere takes place with the patient in the normal state of consciousness, and to all intents and purposes can be considered as a more extended form of a normal medical interview.

The analysis of the non-verbal, emotional hemisphere is undertaken in the altered state of consciousness we recognize as the hypnotic state.

In the normal (verbal) state of consciousness the left hemisphere is dominant, and if it finds it necessary to clothe a word with an emotional overtone it orders the right hemisphere to add an overtone chosen by itself; that is, the left hemisphere. This is rather like selecting a colour from a box of paints to give more substance to a black and white sketch, the box of paints being merely a source of colour and having no influence on the choice. The result is a correct, emotionally embellished, verbal description of the left hemisphere's notion of the subject which, nevertheless, need not correspond to the right hemisphere's ideas on the same subject.

Under hypnosis, the right hemisphere is dominant, and, if it wishes to use words to express itself, then it uses the left hemisphere's vocabulary like a dictionary, but the emotional expression it gives to the words is the true reflection of its own philosophy, which may differ from that of the left.

Occasionally, however, while interviewing a patient in the normal, verbal state of consciousness, a distinct change can be seen to come over the patient's appearance and the patient seems lost in his or her thoughts. This 'wandering off' phenomenon may mean that the patient has changed hemispheres, and that the right is now dominant. If this is true, then it is as if he or she were in an hypnotic state and their emotional behaviour will reflect this hemisphere rather than the verbal hemisphere.

This possibility should be noted, as it may affect the analysis. For example, a patient of mine, when verbally describing his own reaction to his father's behaviour towards him, showed considerable sympathy for the attitude his father had adopted. However, at one point in my patient's narrative his speech slowed and his face took on a vacant look, the tone of his voice altered into an angry note, and he condemned his father's behaviour, saying that he should have known better. He then suddenly seemed to snap out of this state, apologized for this opinion, and continued to support his father. It subsequently turned out that he was indeed at emotional loggerheads with his father, but at the same time he had logically to agree with the correctness of his father's attitude. I am quite sure that this momentary change was a true expression of the right hemisphere's feelings on the subject and was the first glimpse of the conflict I needed to resolve.

In the case of Mrs X, however, her verbal description of the hospital scene, although punctuated at times by a non-verbal description, was not in conflict with the latter and led me to believe that this traumatic event was not the source of her presenting symptoms. This view was supported by the verbal answer she gave to my questions on the importance of the incident to her life. The general gist of her answer was that it had indeed affected her profoundly in many ways. She realized that it could have been just as easily her in that hospital bed. It altered her whole outlook on riding; she became more careful and her riding suffered for quite some time.

The sight of Jane looking as she did was such a shock to Susan that she felt she aged years in those few minutes. It also impressed her with her own good fortune, and she realized she was a privileged individual in a cruel world. She ended, 'And I am constantly reminded of Jane, those wretched pandas crop up all over the place!'

However, Mrs X was certain that her panic attacks were in no way related to Jane's accident. She felt that the emotions were totally different; whereas one was of shock, horror, then sadness, the other was of fear.

I accepted this explanation when she offered it because it fitted in with the observations I have just described.

So far, then, the verbal analysis of my patient's childhood and adolescence had revealed no obvious evidence of an interhemispheric conflict of such a major nature that one could suspect it as a source or cause of her panic attacks. Perhaps I was wrong; perhaps I had missed something that would reveal its importance when the right hemisphere was analysed under hypnosis. This occurs not infrequently. The verbal description of an episode in a patient's life is often described with such disarming nonchalance that it is overlooked until age regression displays its true significance. If this was so I would have to wait. In the meanwhile, let me proceed with Mrs X's verbal description of her adult life from the age of eighteen to the point at which she consulted me.

From her coming of age at eighteen to her marriage at twenty-four, Susan enjoyed an active social life. She engaged in the usual round of parties, throwing the odd one or two herself. She learnt to control her alcohol intake after suffering from an over-indulgence which had exposed a certain vulnerability – she tended to become amorous when drunk, then regretted it later! It was after one such occasion, which had ended by her having to fight off some of the more demanding attentions of a male guest, that she decided it was about time she lost her virginity and gained some positive sexual experience with someone she really liked.

She came to the conclusion that it would be far better to organize this 'event' in as calculating a way as possible, rather than risk a sordid affair on a couch at a party with someone she barely knew and who would probably be half drunk to boot!

It must be pointed out that at no time in her life up to then had Susan been 'in love', as it were, although she acknowledged having crushes on various unobtainable males since the age of twelve. In particular, she remembers a master at school who was the idol of many of the girls, and a riding instructor who was more personally 'hers'. Neither of these individuals were ever aware of her feelings; she used them merely as real figures on which to base her fantasy lovers. It was interesting that the schoolmaster tended to enter her fantasies in a kindly, encouraging, asexual way, whereas the riding instructor was unquestionably a seducer.

At the age of eighteen it was noticeable that she preferred the company of older men rather than her own immediate age group; whom she considered gauche and often childish. As an only child she had been used to adults around her, and this was repeated in her riding environment, where children were in a minority; such children as were there tended to be a dedicated and responsible bunch intent on learning from their elders and betters.

When Susan organized her 'big event', as she put it, her partner was, not surprisingly, eight years her senior and married. Mrs Susan X's light-hearted account of this important episode in her life was most amusing.

Her very first words as she began her recollection were, 'I don't know how I dared to do it!' and were accompanied by a ripple of laughter, bouts of which were to occur again and again as she unfolded her Canterbury tale. The fact that she did dare exposed an important pattern of behaviour, which became more significant later in exploring the origin of her panic attacks.

As I have previously mentioned, Susan left school at the age of eighteen to work in her father's business. She worked hard and with enthusiasm and was always one of the last to leave the office. She knew that nepotism could be a criticism, and she was determined to earn her position in the firm by her own efforts rather than by being the 'boss's daughter'.

Her organizing ability was soon recognized, which led her to gravitate to the expansion side of the business, where this talent was put to good use. She soon became an important part of the team involved in searching for suitable sites for petrol filling-stations, their purchase with planning permission and eventual construction. The job involved travelling widely and meeting numerous individuals; these included the owners of the property to be purchased, local officials in the various planning offices, oil company representatives, architects, builders and so on. Her father led this team, and was delighted with the easy manner his daughter exhibited with their clients as well as her rapid grasp of the correct choice of sites. He also noticed for the first time how valuable the presence of an attractive female can be in business transactions. He remarked on one occasion how people he had previously considered difficult and obstructive altered in the presence of his daughter and became affable and constructive. As time progressed he was able to delegate more and more of this side of his business to his daughter, reducing his control to an advisory capacity and releasing time for himself to attend to other parts of his business.

In the course of this work Susan had met, on several occasions, the retail business representative of a well-known oil company. This company's franchise was much sort after; their products were household names and sales of them were guaranteed. Whenever a suitable site for a petrol station was obtained it was this company's brand of petrol that was given first consideration.

Frequently, however, this company was unable to grant a franchise because of the proximity of another petrol station already selling their brand. Despite this etiquette, it was possible to persuade the company to change its allegiance if it could be shown that the new site was far superior to the already existing petrol station. Although gallonage of petrol sold was of prime importance, other factors such as ease and safety of entrance to and exits from the pumps, space available for lubrication bays and car washes and so on, could all be points favouring the new site over any loyalty to the existing one.

Susan, in a hard-hitting campaign, had successfully persuaded this company that her site was superior to that of a rival station already in existence. It was during the lengthy negotiations leading to this decision that Susan had become well acquainted with their representative, and she had found him amusing and attractive.

Walter Schroeder was a tall, blond South African with a degree in science from the University of Witwatersrand. His father was already in a high position in the South African division of this multi-national petroleum company, and there was no doubt that his son was being groomed by the company to occupy a similar position. Susan had discovered that Mr Schroeder had been married two years and that his wife was a university lecturer. He had recently spent six months in Germany, throughout which time he had been accompanied by his wife. His English appointment was for one year only, after which he was to be six months in Holland, then three years in America. His wife had returned to her university post in South Africa after their sojourn in Germany and was to remain there until her husband transferred to America. She had already organized a research post in an American university in order to continue with her career.

The twenty-seven-year-old South African obviously enjoyed the presence of women and was particularly attentive to Susan. At one of their meetings he casually invited her up to London for the week-end but, seeing a quizzical look come over Susan's face, he hastily added, 'Oh my wife would not mind, we have a special agreement to cover this year!' Susan dismissed the remark with a light laugh but made a mental note that he was hers for the asking, albeit only on a temporary loan!

Mr Schroeder's petroleum company held an annual trade fair at which it exhibited all the latest machinery associated with petrol stations along with various products for retail sale. It also announced its yearly promotions and future advertising campaigns in the press and on television. Owners of petrol stations were offered free overnight accommodation at local hotels of their choice, and the exhibition usually lasted from midday on a Friday until 5.00 p.m. the next day.

Walter – he insisted on the use of his first name – had made a point of reminding Susan of this event and hoped to see her there with her father. Susan's father, however, rarely attended such functions, considering them a waste of time and just an excuse by a multi-national company to spend money which would otherwise have gone to the host government. He thought that Susan was of the same mind, and was surprised when she volunteered to take up the invitation as representative of their own company. 'Do you really want to go?' he asked. 'Yes', she replied, 'it is being held this year in Canterbury and it is an excellent opportunity to have a good look at the city and cathedral. We have only ever passed through on our way to Dover which is a pity because it has always looked so attractive.' She meant this, although admitted to herself an ulterior motive.

When the usual invitation arrived Susan replied, accepting for herself, but instead of sending it to the course organizer, she included it in the envelope of a letter concerning the development of a new site and addressed personally to Mr Schroeder.

She added a postscript in her own handwriting – 'Please pass on the enclosed' – as if it were an afterthought. She now knew that he would be aware of the hotel at which she would be staying and what is more that she would be on her own.

Three days later Susan received an entrance pass to the trade fair, a confirmation of a single-room booking at the Swan Hotel, a lapel badge with her printed name and a handwritten note from Walter asking her to dine with him on the Friday evening.

The occasion turned out to be an even greater success than Susan had hoped. The weather was sunny and warm, Canterbury was a medieval joy to explore, even the trade fair was interesting. Walter had chosen an expensive and exclusive country club at which to dine, and his manners and attention were impeccable throughout the evening. On the way back to her hotel he drew up his Mercedes outside an old, fifteenth-century coaching inn, and over a gin and tonic confessed that he was staying at the same hotel as she was and that he had seen to it that they were the only two from the trade fair that had been booked in by the petroleum company. She thanked him and kissed him. Later, as she stepped into the car, her skirt caught up and exposed a length of thigh, she left her skirt unadjusted. By the time they reached his room in the Swan it was hardly necessary to open the iced champagne he had previously ordered, but it was another nice touch, Susan thought, before her senses overwhelmed her and she more than willingly assisted in the loss of her virginity.

Admittedly, there was a certain amount of emotion associated with the aftermath of Canterbury. Susan felt a different individual in some ways and she knew, were the affair to continue, she could become vulnerable. Walter was insistent that they saw each other again, but Susan had no illusions about his motives.

He was a sexual man temporarily devoid of a natural outlet. He would never stoop to an English prostitute and his only remedy was an English mistress, preferably unencumbered. It was much to his credit, Susan thought, that he had never denied this fact, and discussions had occurred between them quite openly on these lines.

The problem, if it was a problem for Susan, resolved itself quite dramatically. Walter was suddenly recalled to South Africa by his family after his father suffered a severe stroke and was not expected to live.

Susan saw him fleetingly for a few hours in London before he boarded a flight to Johannesburg. She never saw him again. His career followed the predicted course and he is now a chief executive of the company in South Africa.

Some weeks following Walter's departure Susan was introduced, at a party, to Mr Geoffrey X, whom later she was to marry. Geoffrey apparently fell in love with Susan as soon as he saw her. For Susan it was a much more gradual process but equally positive.

Geoffrey was a tall, dark, good-looking introvert, who exhibited a definite shyness towards women. He was three years older than Susan and was the most junior in a firm of solicitors working in the City. He was specializing in international law and hoped eventually to set up his own consultancy in this field.

Geoffrey had a younger brother, James, with whom he shared a large flat in South Kensington. James was mad on flying and was training with British Airways to be an airline pilot. Although looking like a smaller edition of his elder brother, James was a completely different character, a fun-loving extrovert fond of all varieties of sport, and he had a reputation with women. Their parents, well-to-do hoteliers, had sent them both to the same public school.

Despite their differences in character, or possibly because of them, the two brothers got on very well with each other, respecting each other's private lives and never interfering in them. Geoffrey's life was well regulated whereas James's was not, and, apart from the odd game of squash they played together, they led very separate social lives and rarely met. The first time Susan saw the two brothers together was at her engagement party with Geoffrey, when James, true to form, enlivened the proceedings with a certain amount of outrageous behaviour, which ended up with a strip-tease greatly egged on by Pamela, who later disappeared with him to a night-club.

Susan married Geoffrey in May 1966. It was a splendid wedding, both sets of friends fitting in well with each other, aided no doubt by unlimited champagne at the lavish reception – a good start to a marriage which had the possibility of a lasting potential.

However, an incident did occur, after the first year of their marriage, which could have been disastrous. Susan knew that at some point in her medical history she would have to discuss this incident with me and was always prepared to do so, but it did involve her in a moral dilemma.

She had evidently entered into a mutual promise never to reveal the incident nor to divulge the name of the male individual concerned because of the unnecessary damage that would ensue to the respective families involved. It was this promise that had worried her. Typically, she compromised, and in an obviously prepared little speech she asked me if she could discuss the incident but withhold the identity of the individual.

To me, of course, this was a verbal censorship. The left hemisphere was laying down the rules as to the degree of honesty it was prepared to allow. I strongly suspected that there would be more than just a name censored. The name really did not matter; what was important was the right hemisphere's description of the episode, and that could come out under hypnosis. I was prepared to wait. I accepted her conditions.

Susan took my acceptance with a nod and a smile as if she knew it was the obvious reply; there was no sign of any emotion as she quietly spoke.

Some time after my marriage I was raped by a friend of my husband's family whom I hardly knew. The whole episode was so sudden that I was completely taken by surprise. We had thrown a party and this man's girlfriend, who was not used to drink, became very ill and started to be sick. He and I helped her upstairs to the bathroom followed by a few others in the party. I shooed them all off saying that the two of us would cope with her and that they were to rejoin the party. We coped as well as we could with her in the bathroom but at one point she vomited straight into my lap and the rest went over her boy-friend's trousers. My dress was drenched and it was soaking through to my pants; his trousers were spattered all over.

I told him to take off his trousers and chuck them in the bath and that I would lend him a pair of my husband's shorts; at the same time I took off my dress and pants and dumped them in the bath with his. I put a towel around my waist and cleaned myself up. He, in his underpants and shirt, attended to his girlfriend, who was sobering up, then the both of us in this strange attire helped her along to a spare bedroom where we left her on the bed to recover. I told him to wait whilst I brought him some shorts. As I returned along the corridor with the shorts a hand grasped me and I was pulled into the darkness of an adjacent bedroom.

At first I thought he was just fooling but I soon realized he was naked and very excited. My mind was in a total whirl. I just could not think of what to do and I seemed to be struck dumb, no words would come. He pushed me onto the bed and for some extraordinary reason I did not seem to resist. Before I had time to recover my thoughts from the shock and sheer speed of the attack, he was having intercourse with me.

I suppose one must call it rape. It was a total surprise. I would never have allowed it to happen under normal circumstances. As it was, to my everlasting shame, I had an orgasm within seconds of him entering me. Because of this I had an over-whelming feeling of guilt which took away the anger I should have felt towards his behaviour. I suppose the whole incident took about three minutes.

We tidied ourselves up, I put on another dress, and we joined the party again, no words had passed between us: everybody was sympathetic about my clothes but were very amused at his shorts.

He telephoned me early the next day full of remorse. By this time the full implications of the incident had hit us both very hard and I wanted to discuss the matter with him. We met in a local coffee-room where he apologized for his behaviour and thanked me for my discretion.

We mutually agreed that we would both completely forget the incident and gave each other solemn promises never to divulge the episode.

I believed her. I could see no reason why she should lie. Her promise was a sufficient excuse for her to withhold the identity of the man.

I questioned her as to whether she felt the incident had anything to do with her panic attacks, and her verbally emphatic answer was 'No!' She said that as the incident was well over two years ago, she would have expected any panic attacks to have started at the time it occurred, or at least soon afterwards. As far as she was concerned her guilt was resolved after the conversation in the coffee-room the following morning and she blamed the influence of alcohol on being the prime cause of initiating his, and then subsequently her, behaviour.

Before completing the verbal analysis of this patient's adult life I wanted to make sure of the left hemisphere's opinion on certain moral values, particularly if these in any way seemed to clash with her emotional behaviour.

I questioned her first of all on the influence of her grandfather. He was a Methodist minister. Was he morally aggressive about his beliefs? Did he demand a belief in God, and did he expect a belief in God in all the members of his family?

Her answer was interesting. Yes, he firmly believed in God as portrayed by the New Testament but he was definitely not morally aggressive and never demanded loyalty to his beliefs from his family. His philosophy was such that it was up to the individuals to listen to 'the Word' and make up their own minds.

What was his attitude to divorce? He deplored that any marriage should ever come to the stage of even contemplating divorce but accepted that couples often marry for the wrong reasons and that people's feelings can change in the course of their lives. If a marriage had broken down irrevocably the only answer was divorce, and under those circumstances it was just as much God's will to end it as it was to have brought the couple together in the first place.

In view of this answer, I asked Susan what she thought her grandfather's reaction would have been had he known of her seduction of Walter – a married man. Without any hesitation she replied that he would have been appalled! But after a few moments' contemplation she modified the remark by saying that her grandfather was very much a thinker and would have looked for an explanation. She felt that he would have considered the important factor to be Walter's moral responsibility to his wife, a factor that

Walter and his wife had previously discussed together, and reached a mutually acceptable decision. Nevertheless, he would not have agreed with their conclusion.

I asked Susan if she could have told her grandfather about the affair with Walter? Her answer was 'Good God, No!'

Could she have told her mother? 'Yes, but I would have hated to do so!'

What about her father? 'Oh yes, he would have been amused and probably made some frightful Army-style remark! He would have approved of the choice you see, whereas had it been another person he would probably have been very angry!'

Did she in fact tell her father? 'No! I did not! and, what is more, never will! but I have a little suspicion that he knew about it at the time. He is no fool.'

I took up her mention of 'another person' who would have antagonized her father under such circumstances. It appeared that he was a clerk in her father's office who had a terrible crush on her. She supposed she was flattered, but although she never encouraged him she never really choked him off. His obvious infatuation annoyed her father, who was relieved when this person left for another job.

Finally I came to Susan's own verbal description of her panic attacks.

> I was sitting on the sofa with my husband, it was about seven in the evening and we were watching a news programme on the television. I suddenly felt awful, as if something terrible was going to happen. My heart started beating rapidly and I started trembling all over, I felt very frightened and thought I was going to die. I gripped my husband's arm and said something like 'I feel terrified, don't go away!' Evidently I was as white as a sheet. He cuddled me and gradually the awful feeling went off. Five minutes later I was as right as rain! The next attack occurred a week later. I was by myself in the kitchen making some pastry and feeling perfectly normal when again, quite out of the blue, this sensation of impending doom came over me and my hands started shaking so much that I could no longer roll the pastry.
>
> I felt terrified that this time I really was going to die and I came out in a cold sweat. I sat down in a chair and gradually the fear died away and within five minutes I was to all intents and

purposes back to normal! Since then I have had many more attacks, sometimes two in one day. They always follow the same pattern, coming out of the blue with no obvious reason, and after about three minutes of what is to me a feeling of intense terror, start fading slowly away. Unfortunately they now seem to be affecting me more afterwards. I feel quite weak for an hour or so and I am now becoming very apprehensive of further attacks. One way or another it is affecting my whole life, but strangely enough, to my doctor's surprise, I do not feel unduly depressed. I wish they would go. I have this feeling that if I only knew what I was frightened of I would be able to overcome it somehow. The doctors tell me that they can find nothing physically wrong with me, which is very reassuring in one way but does not solve the problem of why I am having them, and why me?

I felt that the verbal hemisphere analysis of Mrs Susan X was as complete as was necessary and that I should now move on to compare this view with that of her emotional hemisphere.

In all the treatment sessions so far, the hour of appointment time had been taken up by 45 minutes of verbal interview and a final 15 minutes with the patient *relaxing in the hypnotic state*. The patient sits in a comfortable armchair and I sit beside her on her right. I give verbal instructions for her to follow, which enables her to enter into the hypnotic state. There is no eye-contact. This is my standard procedure and, until I am satisfied with the verbal analysis, I make no attempt to unravel any emotional events under hypnosis. There are several important reasons for adopting this technique.

First of all, it introduces patients to this altered state of consciousness knowing that no demands will be made on them. They are merely to relax and to savour the profound feeling of total lack of tension that hypnosis engenders in both body and mind.

Another effect is to allay any pre-formed fears patients may have about hypnosis – fears often irrational and the result of misleading opinions, superstitions and old wives' tales, gathered at random over the course of their lives. Once these fears are overcome, the patient readily and easily goes into the hypnotic state and achieves a good depth.

This very feeling of peace, tranquillity and total freedom from all tension experienced by patients in hypnosis is therapeutic in its own right, and they look forward to entering into this state again.

The only form of treatment given during this 15 minutes is one of ego-strengthening in which the confidence of the patient in the ability to overcome any problem is encouraged, along with a more positive re-alignment of the patient's self-image. In experiencing this altered state of consciousness patients are aware that something profound is happening to them, which tends to increase their support for the treatment and diminish the doubts.

I am often quite surprised by the improvement in the patient's condition as a result of this simple form of therapy under hypnosis. Mrs X was no exception, and already at this point in her treatment had noticed a diminution in the strength and frequency of her panic attacks.

The method's main purpose, however, is to prepare the patient for the emotional exposure necessary to reveal underlying inter-hemispheric discrepancies.

In the several hour-long sessions under hypnosis that followed, Mrs X was taken back into the various incidents in her life that could have had some bearing on the cause of her presenting symptom.

Her early childhood was re-enacted in detail, with emphasis on the role played by her grandparents; her schooldays; her attitude to her mother and father; the thrills and fears of her riding successes and failures.

Attention was focused on her emotional involvement with her school-friends and her riding circle, Pamela in particular.

Later, the years working with her father as boss, and her re-lationship to him, were considered; also her attitude and expec-tations of any male behaviour she experienced; finally, her own marriage and the birth of her son.

The nearest to any form of emotional abreaction occurring in the course of these sessions was in the recall of the Jane episode, but even this was very short-lived, and was in response to a feeling of sadness for Jane rather than a personal anxiety.

The breakthrough came when we tackled the occurrence of her first panic attack. In a deep hypnotic state she was asked to go back in time to this first attack. She was asked to see herself there with her husband watching a 'current affairs programme' (I quoted from her doctor's letter) on the television. As soon as she felt that she was really there in time and place she was to signal to me by raising the index finger of her left hand.

She never signalled. A period elapsed in which no movement occurred, then a slow smile appeared over her face and her arms started to move upwards; she looked as if she was throwing something like a ball at a coconut-shy. These movements with her arms continued for some time and her breathing became quite rapid. They ended with her falling back in the chair with her legs in an extended position and rigid as if in a fit. Very slowly the muscles relaxed, her breathing calmed and her body went totally limp. As it did so, her eyes opened and she stared unseeingly at the ceiling for a while before they closed again.

The abreaction was over.

My usual method of terminating the hypnotic state is to tell the patient that I will count up to twenty, during which time they will return to their normal, conscious self. This I did, adding that she would remember every incident that had occurred in the session and would be able to describe and freely discuss it with me.

Returning to normal consciousness after a deep hypnotic state should not be hurried. Even after the eyes have opened, the muscle-tone has returned, and the body readjusted itself in the chair, the patient may still appear to be in a slight daze. While in this state Mrs X slowly moved her hand to her forehead and felt a forelock of her hair. She then looked at her hand as if she expected to see something on it. Seeing nothing, she then felt under her chin and then looked down at her dress. Seemingly satisfied that nothing was amiss, the dazed look disappeared and she turned to me with a wan smile.

I waited patiently for her explanation of the session's events.

Nothing was forthcoming. During a long period of silence she turned her head towards me on two occasions as if about to speak, then seemed to think better of it and turned her head away again.

Eventually she said very slowly, 'Do you mind if I go now, I have a lot to think about.' It was not a request; it was a statement, and the quiet determination in her voice signalled to me that to press for a discussion would be therapeutically unwise at this stage.

I said, 'Of course!' and moved over to the door to open it for her. As she rose from the chair she looked closely at her dress as if to make sure there was nothing out of place. In passing me she paused and said, 'Thank you, I believe I have just learnt something about myself of importance but at the moment I do not feel able to discuss it.' Her voice was quite different, businesslike and confident.

Further appointments are made by my secretary as the patient leaves. Mrs X declined the offer on this occasion saying that she would telephone later after she had consulted her diary.

Over a week went by before she contacted my secretary, and then it was only to say that she was taking a short holiday with her husband and would telephone on her return. No mention was made of her panic attacks.

Some three weeks after her last appointment Mrs X telephoned me personally. The gist of the conversation was that she had suffered no further panic attacks since our last meeting, that she was feeling much more confident in herself and that she saw no need for any further appointments as long as this state of affairs continued.

I countered by saying that although I was delighted with her improvement it was important at some stage for her to discuss her abreaction with me and not just to break off at this point. She agreed with this, and I had the feeling that she would have liked to have discussed everything with me but something was holding her back – it was a 'something' she had to work out herself and not for me to force.

I have frequently found, when age-regressing patients under hypnosis, they have subsequently voiced surprise at the detailed visual memory of the scenes they were reviewing and the emotions that accompanied the scenes. For instance, one patient of mine was regressed to an incident in her early childhood when her mother announced to her brother and herself that their father had left them to live with another woman.

This patient felt a sudden feeling of hate surge up in her against her mother. She felt her mother was the cause of her father's departure, a feeling she had never, to her knowledge, previously entertained. In fact, quite to the contrary, she had always felt extremely sorry for her mother and considered her father to have let them all down disgracefully!

The surprise and strength of this new emotion gave the patient quite a shock; she felt embarrassed and found it difficult to discuss. When she eventually did manage to talk about it she experienced a deep sense of relief.

I felt something similar had occurred in Mrs X's mind and that sooner or later she would be able to overcome any embarrassment she might have in disclosing it to me.

I was quite wrong. There had been no embarrassment; it was more a revelation that had occurred during the hypnotic session; a realization that had set her a very difficult problem!

True to form, Susan X set about the task as calculatingly as her 'Canterbury tale'. When, some weeks later, she made an appointment to see me she had already made up her mind on the steps necessary to solve the problem.

All she needed from me, it would turn out, was an approval.

When Susan entered the room her mood was apologetic but confident.

She started off with, 'I am sorry if I have appeared rude in ignoring you over the past weeks but in truth I have not. Several times I have had an almost irresistible urge to telephone you for an appointment but have decided against doing so before I was certain of my facts.'

With these remarks she seated herself in the chair in front of my desk and put her bag down on the floor near her feet. I had hardly seated myself before Mrs X continued.

'I no longer need any treatment but I would be very grateful for your advice and understanding.'

I reassured her that I would do my best. Seemingly satisfied with this, she relaxed back in the chair and commenced to explain the events that had stemmed from our last treatment session. Her words were:

'As was usual I felt very relaxed and pleasantly warm as I drifted off into the hypnotic state. Then you asked me to go back in time to the point of the first panic attack. I did so and visualized myself at home watching television. I felt fine. Then 'you said to me – "you are watching a current affairs programme" – and immediately on hearing these words I started to feel panicky. You then followed up with, "As soon as you really feel you are there just raise the index finger of your left hand". As you said these words the scene seemed to change and I was in my bedroom, in my dressing-gown, and about to have a bath. The panicky feeling had gone.'

Mrs X stopped at this point, took in a deep breath, smiled somewhat grimly, then snapped, 'Now for the confession!' She paused and looked at me as if expecting some reaction, then continued.

'You remember I described to you a sort of rape I experienced some time after I had been married?'

I nodded.

She went on.

Everything that occurred to me was a true and exact description of what happened on that occasion. His girlfriend was sick over the both of us and we had to change our clothes. On the way back from getting him a change of trousers he grabbed me, pulled me into the spare bedroom, and tried to rape me . . . But in fact he did not get anywhere near me! I hit him hard across the face and he stopped in his tracks! I was furious! I told him to leave, along with his girlfriend, as soon as she was in a fit condition.

It is true that he did telephone me the next day. I did meet him over a coffee; he did apologize, blaming the drink: I did agree to forget the incident but no promises were made, and there is another point. This whole incident occurred before I was married and before I had even met my husband!

Mrs X paused again, and I must have moved as if to speak because she hurriedly carried on with: 'No questions yet, let me finish!' So she continued:

I have actually combined two incidents. Both descriptions are accurate. The first ends with the slapped face, the second starts just before that happened, and occurred when I was married. The first involved Tony Best, a young man in a group of us who were friends at that time, and took place at a party I gave at my parents' home; the second involved an unmarried associate of my husband who was staying the night with us before moving on the next day to London. It was with this man that I made the mutual promise never to divulge the incident or his name, and as you now know I went to elaborate lengths to disguise him.

Now, at my last treatment session, I had a clear vision of the second incident, and in seeing it again I suddenly realized something that had never occurred to me before! I have spent the last few weeks verifying some facts. The result is I feel that I must now put these facts to you, explain what I intend to do, and seek your approval.

To do this I must give you an unexpurgated description of this second incident!

Her last few words were accompanied by a disarming chuckle and a wide smile. She then went on to say.

As I said previously, this man was staying overnight with us and was due to catch the midday train back to London.

My husband left for work as usual at 8.00 a.m. and I prepared to get on with the day by taking a bath. I was in the bathroom running the water for my bath and had removed my dressing gown. I did not hear the door open because of the noise of the water. The first I knew of his presence was the slap of a cold-watered flannel as it hit my back.

He had aimed it at me from just outside the door, then, laughing all the time, he retreated along the corridor.

The cold water stung me into action. I picked up the flannel and hurled it back at him but he dodged into his room and it missed him. I hastily put on my dressing gown, picked up the flannel again and burst into his room to do battle. Thereupon there followed a certain amount of horse-play, which included an exhausting pillow-fight. Eventually, and quite out of breath, I called a truce and sat down on the edge of his bed.

My hair was in total disarray, my dressing-gown had become untied exposing the front of my body, and I was naked underneath.

As I recovered my breath I suddenly became aware of this and realized he must be looking at me. I slowly raised my head to look at him. He was standing a few feet away with his back toward me. He had slipped his dressing-gown off which lay crumpled at his feet.

He was naked.

He turned round slowly to face me.

His penis was hugely erect.

I became rooted to the spot and remember blushing scarlet. He moved over to me and gently pushed me back on to the bed. I seemed totally unable to resist or even speak. He moved my legs apart and lowered himself on top of me.

I felt him enter me.

The amazing thing was that I was wide open to accept him! A thing that had never happened to me with any man before in my life! In the usual run of events I need quite a long session of physical foreplay and, more often than not, my husband will use a lubricant. Furthermore, within a few seconds of him entering me I had the most colossal orgasm I had ever experienced, and what is more I had several of them before I felt his penis swell and thrust harder as he approached his climax.

This point was terrible because he withdrew suddenly and I hated it, I even tried desperately to hold him inside me but he was too strong. As he withdrew, his semen squirted out of his penis with such force that some of it landed on my forehead and hair, some under my chin and between my breasts, and, as he continued to pump it out, a pool of it collected in my navel and trickled down either side of my body. There seemed to be a tremendous amount of it and it was streaked with a white substance. I was obviously fascinated by it because normally I would take very little notice of such a happening and I put it down to the extreme sexual high I was experiencing.

We had almost continuous intercourse for the next *three hours* and I maintained throughout this time a huge sexual plateau which produced multiple orgasmic peaks. There was no doubt that I had been awakened sexually for the very first time and I was very grateful for it.

Before the man left we had a discussion and we both decided that we would totally forget the incident and, as you know, we made a solemn promise never to divulge it to anyone!

He only just caught his train!

The next day was peculiar. I had very mixed feelings, which were not helped by the onset of my period. Certainly I had some remorse, but as time went by, and I was able to actually repeat the peak of sexual feeling with my husband, I came to look upon the incident as heaven-sent rather than sordid, particularly as it was soon after that that I managed to become pregnant and I felt certain this was due to my heightened sexuality and the increase in the number and strength of the orgasms I was able to achieve.

Mrs X paused and I was able to ask her if she had continued to see this man.

She replied that if I meant 'have intercourse with him' then the answer was 'NEVER', but she had seen him on several occasions because circumstances were such that it was impossible for her not to do so.

Mrs Susan X then proceeded to relate a most extraordinary tale.

'Now let me return to that last treatment session,' she said.

You remember I first felt panicky, then this passed off as the scene changed to me running a bath? That scene, as you may have already guessed, was a total re-run of the events I have just described. I was there again, I totally re-lived every minute of it in exact detail, the flannel, the pillow-fight, the intercourse, everything, until he ejaculated all over me and I found myself in a sexual turmoil staring at the sight and quantity of his semen.

Then everything seemed to freeze and stop, and it suddenly occurred to me that my husband's semen looked nothing like this, nor had I ever seen him ejaculate anything like that amount!

It was a shock! Then I heard you counting and I slowly came back to reality – or at least what I thought was reality – but, unlike other times, I still felt in a daze and my mind was a whirl of thoughts.

I couldn't make it out at first but it gradually began to dawn on me that my husband's semen may not be up to scratch. I had often heard of men with low sperm counts and perhaps this was why it took me so long to get pregnant in the first place. Perhaps it was also the cause of the failure of our present attempts for our second baby. As these thoughts took place I began to feel a whole lot better, almost elated. If this really was the cause of my failure to get pregnant then surely it should be easy, either to treat my husband, or to store his semen until there was enough of the stuff to impregnate me. Then I became depressed as a little voice seemed to say that I was thinking a load of nonsense. But I could not get the idea out of my mind and I became determined to investigate this possible explanation.

I was by now fully in control of myself but really did not feel up to discussing the session and, as you know, I left fairly abruptly. The next couple of hours were probably the most thoughtful I had ever spent.

One of the questions I had to ask myself was how I was to approach my husband on this matter. This was probably the most difficult problem I had to face, although at the time I just felt like telephoning him as soon as I returned home! Fortunately, the train journey gave me time to reflect a little and by the time the journey ended I had decided to say nothing at all to him until I had thought about it a little more and perhaps sought some professional advice. In addition, I was in a peculiar mood, elated but relaxed. I felt confident in myself again, a thing that had been lacking since the onset of my panic attacks. I felt that at last I had something substantial, something I could get my teeth into, almost like being back at work with an interesting problem to solve. I was sexually disturbed. The reality of the remembered experience was as vivid as if it had occurred for the first time. It had released again the myriad of thoughts and emotions associated with that astonishing day and I revelled in my day-dreaming.

The next day I set about the task in earnest. I decided that this was not a problem in which you should be involved, at least, not at this stage, although I did seriously consider it for quite some time. Instead I telephoned a school-friend of mine who had taken up medicine and was now a qualified doctor working in a hospital. We had not seen each other for some time and she was delighted to meet me for lunch at an hotel near her hospital. Over the telephone I had told her that I had a small problem and would be very grateful for her advice, so after exhausting all the gossip concerning our mutual friends, including ourselves, we took coffee in a secluded part of the lounge and I launched into my prepared story. Very briefly it was that I was slow to become pregnant with my first child, that the same thing was happening again with the attempt at the second, that I appeared to be normal according to my GP, which left the possibility of a husband with a low fertility.

My husband knew nothing of my fears; after all, we had one child, and presumably it was only a matter of time and persever-ance before I was pregnant again (I never mentioned anything about panic attacks).

Was it possible, were I to obtain some of my husband's semen, to have it analysed without him getting to know the result?

My doctor friend asked, 'Why the secrecy?' I told her that if it turned out that my husband was normal then I would feel an awful fool. On the other hand, were he to have a low count it might affect him psychologically and cause unnecessary worry at a very important time in his career when he was just about to branch out on his own.

My friend supportingly accepted this explanation, and even went on to say that there were many instances of a deterioration of sexual activity in the male following the discovery of a low sperm count, which could only be explained in terms of its being a blow to the male ego. She added that the sperm count had to be pretty low to affect fertility significantly, but agreed with me that, as some men could be very touchy on these matters, it would be better if they did not know, but she could not see how on earth this could be avoided!

This was all I wanted. I explained that whenever my husband used a condom I was always the one that ended up with removing it from his deflated penis to avoid any mess. I usually tied a knot in it, wrapped it in a tissue, and disposed of it later. I must say that she found the thought of my activity in this way highly amusing and could not get over my husband's chauvinism. When her laughter had died down she looked me straight in the face, and said: 'Well, if it is as easy as that, all you have to do is to bring me the goods as soon after intercourse as possible and I will have a count done for you!' She added as an afterthought that I must make sure the french-letter was a plain one and not spermicide-incorporated.

I arranged to deliver the 'goods' personally to her, in a specimen bottle she supplied, at 8.30 the next morning or one of the mornings in the week.

I had no difficulty. As you know, my husband and I had decided soon after the onset of my panic attacks to postpone the idea of another pregnancy until I felt confident enough to tackle it, and in the meanwhile he had gone back to the temporary use of a condom.

My doctor friend telephoned me later in the week and I met her in her room in the hospital. She told me that the result of the test had come back 'azoospermic', which evidently meant that my husband was *totally infertile*!

I simply could not believe it! I had expected a low count, *but no sperms at all* was surely impossible!

My friend saw my confusion and tried to soften the blow by suggesting that the one specimen might not be accurate and proposed that a further two specimens should be examined at weekly intervals. She was clearly upset herself and thought the laboratory might have made a mistake. I sincerely hoped she was right because already certain thoughts had flashed through my mind and I needed to make a few calculations! I agreed to produce the extra evidence and we left it that I should do so over the next three weeks.

In the period of waiting for the results I had to ask myself, if my husband proved to be totally infertile, when had this occurred? The only answer could be – after the birth of our son – unless . . .!

As the second and then the third specimen came back 'azoospermic' the possibility of his not being the parent had to be faced.

My doctor school-friend was simply wonderful about this matter. It had obviously occurred to her, so it came as no surprise when I eventually made the decision to broach her on its medical feasibility.

The only person whom it could possibly have been other than my husband was, of course, the one I have described. But I had a menstrual period after that episode.

She went very carefully into my dates and found to my dismay that the baby was not two weeks premature as was mooted at his birth, but *exactly on time* if our friend was implicated.

She also stated that the period was probably not a true period but a bleed that was the result of some hefty intercourse, an occurrence well known to the medical profession.

I personally have no doubt now that the father of my child is James, my husband's brother.

She dropped this bombshell in a quiet voice but with her head lowered: slowly her face lifted and her eyes contacted mine, and she said: 'I hope this explains my behaviour over the last few weeks.'

These last few words were pathetically inadequate to portray what must have seemed to her an agonizing age of emotional reasoning, calculations and conclusions, and I was impressed with her composure under such circumstances. Here indeed was a woman who was back in control of herself. I felt that I had now only a minor part left to play in her recovery.

The identity of her seducer had taken me by surprise and its implications were immense. At last I fully understood why she had gone to such lengths to disguise this individual! In the conversation that followed I was able to point this out and at the same time agree with her on the absolute necessity for her to have maintained this secrecy. Indeed, I even questioned her reason in revealing his name to me now.

Her answer was another shock!

It is essential for you to know that it was James if you are to be able to give me advice and understanding. Although I have made up my mind about the future, you are the only person I could possibly trust with this knowledge; I suppose, in effect, I am really asking for your blessing on my decisions.

Obviously I have given a tremendous amount of thought about my position.

First of all, I have a husband whom I love and could never harm in any way whatsoever. If I were to reveal all to him I am convinced it would alter, if not ruin, our relationship for the rest of our lives and reflect on our son's happiness. I do not intend ever to tell him.

The second point is that I cannot have any children by my husband. He is very shortly going to question why I cannot. He will demand every possible medical examination and he is bound to find out the reason eventually. He will then deduce that our child is not his. I cannot let this happen!

I have concluded that the only satisfactory path I can take for the well-being of the whole family is to have two more children to complete our original intention.

I intend to seduce James at convenient times in the future to achieve this aim.

It will be easy. My husband is often away for a few days at a time on business, he is usually abroad. James enjoys staying with us and he is company for me in the house. Any children will have a family resemblance and there is no reason why James should suspect that he could be the father. He always applauds my efficiency in all matters and will naturally assume that I am adequately protected with the pill. James, I know, is very fond of me and is always telling me so. In fact his favourite remark, to all and sundry, is that he will only marry when he has found another woman like me!

I have simply no qualms about my decision because I feel that it satisfies every individual concerned without any destruction of the families involved.

I would like you to record this decision in your notes. Were anyone ever to find out, at least my intentions and reasons are there to be revealed if necessary.

She paused, then ended: 'I have made an appointment to see you next week at the same time. I want you to think over my position very carefully just as I have done, I am sure you will come to a similar conclusion. I hope so! I can never thank you enough for all you have done for me.'

With that she left.

Doctors are frequently asked to make far-reaching decisions affecting the lives of their patients and their patients' families. Sometimes this is a relatively easy matter, merely a question of professional knowledge of the malady and producing a statistical answer, for instance, whether it is wise to have a baby immunized against diphtheria and so on.

A decision becomes more difficult where the medical profession itself is divided, as, say, in the treatment of cancer of the breast, where surgical removal or radiotherapy are the alternatives. In such cases even regional differences in treatment patterns should come into consideration.

Where moral questions are involved, complicating factors are quadrupled and it is sometimes impossible to give a truly 'correct' decision. The trap to avoid is producing an answer based purely on the doctor's own moral code without considering that of the patient. A Roman Catholic colleague of mine, who was a gynae-cologist, would give advice to a fellow Catholic only on contracep-tive matters, but he made sure that advice was available in his clinic from experienced doctors holding other faiths. His concern was much appreciated by his staff, the majority of whom were non-Catholics.

But what does one do if it is impossible to pass the buck? My approach in these circumstances is carefully to assess the patient's own attitude to the problem and to try to discern any sign of bias in favour of one decision as opposed to another. If a bias is discovered I would tend to support a decision leaning in this direction even if it was contrary to my own; after all, it is the patient who has to live with the result and not the doctor. For example, an attractive young woman from a wealthy Middle Eastern Muslim family was sent over to a finishing-school in this country. After a year she developed severe migraine, which was put down to the change in climate and food. However, on visits to her parents the migraine attacks increased. Unbeknown to her parents she had met and fallen in love with a young Englishman, who wished to marry her. Her 'headache' was that she knew that this would mean ostracism from her family, whom she loved and deeply respected. Her eventual decision to break off her relationship with the Englishman was very difficult and traumatic but nevertheless the correct one.

Her migraine attacks ceased soon afterwards, which would suggest that the interhemispheric conflict between her moral left and her emotional right hemisphere could have been their cause. The dangers of exposing young men or women at a very vulnerable age to an almost antithetical society in the belief that it is part of their education are not often appreciated. It is unfair to expect them to be immune to the freedoms offered by such societies when no such freedoms exist in their own. They should be well tutored in the pitfalls ahead of them before being subjected to a behavioural norm alien to their upbringing.

In a certain way Mrs Susan X's solution to her problem was outside the behavioural norm of her family – or so it would seem.

She was essentially an honest woman, and I would have thought that she would find it difficult in the long run to sustain such a high degree of pretence. But other factors have to be considered.

Although her moral code was Christian-based, her grandfather, whom she greatly respected, held a very broad view of the faith and it was not unknown for him to adopt an occasional Machiavellian solution to a problem.

Her father was a practical man who had survived a long war mainly in the front-line of activity. He had returned to civilian life with the somewhat cynical philosophy of 'I am all right, Jack', forged out of all the unfairness and anomalies of battle.

Susan herself was a very determined individual who had known where she was going from a very early age. In addition, she was toughly competitive, as shown in her riding successes. She was also a great organizer. It was no secret that one of the major factors in her life's plan was to marry, to have at least three children, and to be part of a happy and successful family. She was well on the way to achieving this when suddenly the earth quaked and she realized her house could crumble. If anyone could pull her plan off it was she; her bias was in favour of trying.

When she took her leave at her last appointment one week later, she was smiling.

I have not seen this patient since, but the last time I heard about her she had three children and was still active in the family business. I can only surmise that she has remained free from further panic attacks.

DISCUSSION OF THE CASE OF MRS SUSAN X IN TERMS OF CAMERAL ANALYSIS

Briefly to reiterate the chapters on theory: in the 1850s Pierre-Paul Broca first alerted the world to the presence of asymmetrical brain-function by showing that part of the speech centre was associated with a distinct area in the left hemisphere. A century later, Roger Sperry and his co-workers dramatically underlined Broca's discovery by their neurological experiments involving the so-called 'split-brain' animals and humans. Since then, an enormous amount of work by many researchers has confirmed the presence of areas in both the left and right hemispheres with specialized and specific functions not duplicated in each hemisphere. Nevertheless, in cases of injury or disease involving a total loss of either the left or the right neocortex, the human individual, although severely incapacitated, is conscious and can continue a meaningful and fulfilling life within human society.

Roger Sperry believes that we are two separate individuals occupying one bony cranium, each with its own interpretation of life's events.

Professor Kinsbourne considers that *bilateral brain symmetry* is programmed only if functional pressures make it necessary; for instance, in turning to the left or the right. For functions unrelated to considerations of symmetry *the brain functions asymmetrically*.

The development of brain asymmetries *in effect* produces a neurological sorting system.

Let me explain this in another way by drawing an analogy with the transmission of a 'Mayday' distress call. Of all the thousands of radio operators listening to their receivers throughout the world, only those tuned into the international distress wavelength will have the knowledge of a distress problem.

Until this message is re-broadcast on other wavelengths or converted for distribution by other communication systems (such as newspapers) it will remain the sole knowledge of the original receivers.

Reaction to the distress signal depends on mobilization of forces capable of solving the distress problem, all of which involve their own communication systems. Supposing the distress call concerned a devastating earthquake in a very remote, mountainous part of the world, and radio signals were too weak for reception to identify the area. Reaction to the devastation would depend on other forms of communication such as seismograph recordings and the aerial pinpointing of the disaster before the problem solving could begin, and thus a delay in this procedure would be inevitable.

Similarly, an emotional message emanating from the limbic system is neurotransmitted equally throughout both cortices but is picked up only by those cells attuned to receive that specific neurotransmitter in the cortex. If it is an emotional problem, it will be the right hemisphere that will pick up the information and initiate problem-solving thought. This can be done both through re-transmitting the information flow and stimulating dynamic interactions between intra- and interhemispheric areas of the brain. Occasionally, as in the earthquake analogy, only indirect information of a problem is available to the cortices and solutions are more difficult to obtain.

In the case of Mrs Susan X, the first *apparent* signal of a serious emotional problem was a panic attack. I feel that this was probably not the first indication, because it was triggered off by a 'current affairs' programme. The pun on the words 'current affairs' was probably the first verbal signal indicating the origin of the problem, because under hypnosis it was these words that appeared to initiate the revealing abreaction.

It is possible that dynamic interhemispheric interaction had already identified a serious emotional problem but was still unaware of its exact nature. More information was still needed. This information was apparently obtained during the abreaction of the so-called rape scene, which alerted the patient to the difference in appearance and amount of the ejaculate compared with that of her husband. If this were so, why had she not noticed it at the time of the original episode? Furthermore, why should she consider the difference in amount and appearance to be necessarily associated with infertility in her husband?

One could argue that, in answer to the first query, she was in such an emotional 'high' that the significance went unnoticed and that it was only on the second re-run, as it were, under hypnosis, that it became obvious. When it comes to the second query it is not quite so straightforward, although the increased amount of ejaculate could be sufficient to suggest inadequacy. Both these answers could explain the source of the missing information necessary for problem-solving dynamic thought. However, I think it interesting to consider even deeper explanations.

It is possible that Mrs X was aware, within months of her marriage, that her husband, although apparently sexually adequate in all respects, had a problem somewhere in this field. Like the weak radio signals from the earthquake zone, the information was insufficient for her to identify the exact area of search until she came to try to get pregnant again.

Science has identified powerful, sexually attracting molecules called pheromones exuded by males and females, which can be picked up by the olfactory nerves in amazingly dilute amounts. Experiments on butterflies have shown that dilutions of one molecule in a square mile is sufficient to guide a sexually potent couple together for mating.

Humans have been shown to excrete these substances, and experiments have been devised to illustrate their influence in, say, a female deciding which seat to sit on in a theatre; she will avoid a seat previously occupied by a female in favour of one previously occupied by a male. The sense of smell is phylogenetically one of the oldest sensory sources of information and is highly developed in primitive reptilia and mammalia. The human race, for a variety of debatable reasons, seems to have lost a lot of its power in this direction; or has it? There is no doubt that humans react to pheromones but are not consciously aware of doing so. Could it be that we have lost or repressed the capability of interpreting the information they provide in the course of evolution? I think it is interesting to consider that the proverbial 'intuition', always held up as a typically feminine attribute, could be women's greater ability to identify pheromones at an unconscious level.

The instinct of the wife to suspect the husband of having a mistress could be that she unconsciously identifies alien pheromones hanging around her husband in a greater strength than usual!

It may be that being 'turned-on' sexually may be initiated by pheromones and could account for extraordinary sexual behaviour exhibited at times between most unlikely people. Susan's profound arousal with James may have been due to her unconscious awareness of his potency compared with that of her husband.

All this, of course, is pure conjecture, but it could help to explain human 'sixth sense' in terms of subliminal information already possessed by the brain from such processes as body-language, chemical messengers, blind sight and so on. To me, these capabilities offer a more acceptable explanation for the apparently inexplicable, and avoid the necessity of having to resort to the fictitious supernatural!

However, the *way* in which differences in knowledge, in interpretation, or actual conflicts arise between the two hemispheres is of relatively little importance; it is the fact that they *exist* that is the paramount factor. Therapeutically they can be revealed by techniques such as age regression, and resolved by re-educative symptom exposure methods and others including abreaction of past emotional events under hypnosis, as in the case of Mrs Susan X.

The medical diagnosis of this case: 'A panic disorder without agoraphobia'.

The *American Diagnostic and Statistical Manual of Mental Disorders III*, revised (DSM 3R) definition of this condition is:

1 Its prevalence is common.
2 Predisposing factors are:
   (a) Separation Anxiety Disorder in childhood;
   (b) sudden loss of social supports;
   (c) disruption of important interpersonal relationships.
3 No organic factors can be established (e.g., thyrotoxicosis).
4 No history of any drug-taking (e.g., caffeine, amphetamines, thyroid).

In Susan X's case the main predisposing factor was the disruption of important interpersonal relationships.

But whatever the method or methods involved, the fact remains that Mrs Susan X became *consciously* aware of a serious problem while under hypnosis.

Notes

Preface

1 MacLean, P.D. (1990) *The Triune Brain in Evolution: Role in Paleo-cerebral Functions*, Plenum Press: New York.
2 Sperry, R.W. (1968) 'Hemisphere deconnection and unity in conscious awareness', *American Psychologist* 23: 723–733.
3 Sperry, R.W., Gazzaniga, M.S. and Bogen, J.E. (1969) 'Interhemispheric relationships: the neocortical commissures: syndromes of hemisphere disconnection', in *Handbook of Clinical Neurology*, P.J. Vinken and G.W. Bruyn (eds) vol 4, Amsterdam: North Holland Publishing Co.
4 Levy, J., Trevarthen, C. and Sperry, R.W. (1972) 'Perception of bilateral chimeric figures following hemispheric deconnection', *Brain* 95: 61–68.

Introduction

1 Farley, J.D. (1976) 'Phylogenetic adaptations and the genetics of psychosis', *Acta Psychiatrica Scandinavica* 53: 173–192.
2 Rollin, H.R. (1991) 'Magic and mountebanks in the development of psychiatric thought', Presidential Address given to the Section of History of Medicine, 1 May 1991 at the Royal Society of Medicine, London.

1   A brief history of hemispheric lateralization

1 Sperry, R.W. (1968) 'Hemispheric deconnection and unity in conscious awareness', *American Psychologist* 23: 723–733.
2 Corballis, M.C. (1980) 'Laterality and myth', *American Psychologist* 35 (3): 284–295.
3 Popper, K.R. and Eccles, J.C. (1977) *The Self and its Brain*, reprinted by Routledge, London and New York, 1990.
4 Tymms, R. (1949) *Doubles in Literary Psychology*, pp. 29, 54–64, 72, 77.

5 Miller, K. (1985) *'Doubles': Studies in Literary History*, Oxford: Oxford University Press.
6 Elliotson, J. (1846) *Harveian Oration*, London: Walton & Mitchell.
7 Wigan, A.L. (1844) *The Duality of the Mind*.
8 Holland, Sir H. (1840) 'On the brain as a double organ', in *Chapters on Mental Physiology*, London: Longman Brown Green & Longman (1852).
9 Myers, F.W. (1885) 'Automatic writing', *Proceedings of the British Society for Psychical Research* 3: 23–63.
10 James, W. (1910) *The Principles of Psychology*, 2 vols.
11 Myers, F.W. (1886) 'Multiplex personality', *The Nineteenth Century* (Nov.): 648–666.
12 Dessoir, M. (1890) *The Double Ego*.
13 Whyte, L.L. (1979) *The Unconscious before Freud*, London: Friedman.
14 Margetts, E.L. (1953) 'Concepts of the unconscious in the history of medical psychology', *Psychiatric Quarterly* 27 (1).
15 Van der Kolk, B.A. and Van der Hart, O. (1989) 'Pierre Janet and the breakdown of adaption in psychological trauma', *American Journal of Psychiatry* 146 (12) (Dec.): 1530–1540.
16 Ellenberger, H.F. (1970) *The Discovery of the Unconscious*, New York: Basic Books
17 James, *Principles of Psychology*.

2 The relationship between hypnosis and the right hemisphere

1 MacLean, P.D. (1955) 'The limbic system ("visceral brain") in relation to central gray and reticulum of the brain-stern. Evidence of interdependence in emotional processes', *Psychosomatic Medicine* 17: 355–366.
2 MacLean, P.D. (1972) 'Cerebral evolution and emotional processes', *Annals of New York Academy of Science* 193: 137.
3 MacLean, P.D. (1976) 'The triune brain – emotion and scientific bias', in *The Neurosciences 2nd Study Programme*, F.O. Schmitt (ed.), New York: Raven Press.
4 MacLean, P.D. (1976) 'Sensory and perceptive factors in emotional functions of the triune brain', in *The Biological Foundation of Psychiatry*, New York: Raven Press.
5 MacLean (1972) 'Cerebral evolution'.
6 Lorenz, K. (1937) 'Uber die Bildung des Instinktbegrieffes', *Naturwissenschaften* 25: 289–300, 307–318, 324–331; also in English translation under the title 'The nature of instinct' in C.H. Schiller (ed.) (1957) *Instinctive Behaviour*, New York: International Universities Press.
7 Tinbergen, N. (1951) *The Study of Instinct*, Oxford: Oxford University Press.
8 Fulton, J.F. (1951) *Frontal Lobectomy and Affective Behaviour*, New York: Norton.
9 MacLean, P.D. (1958) 'The limbic system with respect to self-

preservation and the preservation of the species', *Journal of Nervous and Mental Disorders*, 127: 1.

10 Papez, J.W. (1937) 'A proposed mechanism of emotion', *Archives of Neurology and Psychiatry* 41: 233.

11 Valzelli, L. (1980) 'An approach to neuroanatomical and neurochemical psychophysiology', chap. 1, p. 10, Milan: Edizioni Medico Scientifiche SRL.

12 Kinsbourne, M. (1978) *Asymmetrical Function of the Brain*, Cambridge: Cambridge University Press.

13 Sperry, R.W., Stamm, J.S. and Miner, N. (1956) 'Relearning tests for interocular transfer following division of the optic chiasma and corpus callosum in cats', *Journal of Comparative Physiology and Psychology* 49: 529–533.

14 Bogen, J.E. and Vogel, P.S. (1962) 'Cerebral commissurotomy in man', *Bulletin of the Los Angeles Neurological Society* 29: 169–172.

15 Sperry, R.W. (1968) 'Hemispheric deconnection and unity in conscious awareness', *American Psychologist* 23: 723–733.

16 Gazzaniga, M.S. and Le Doux, J.E. (1978) *The Integrated Mind*, New York: Plenum Press.

17 Wyke, B. (1960) 'Neurological mechanisms in hypnosis: some recent advances in the study of hypnotic phenomena', *Proceedings of the Dental and Medical Society for the Study of Hypnosis* (March): 21.

18 Sperry, R.W. (1968) *Mental Unity Following Surgical Disconnection of the Cerebral Hemispheres*, Harvey Lecture Series 62, New York: Academic Press.

19 Gardner, H. (1977) *The Person after Brain Damage*, London: Routledge & Kegan Paul.

20 Gallwey, W.T. (1974) *The Inner Game of Tennis*, New York: Random House.

21 Edwards, B. (1979) *Drawing on the Right Side of the Brain*, Los Angeles: J.P. Tarcher Inc.

22 Critchley, M. and Henson, R.A. (eds) (1977) *Music and the Brain*, London: Heinemann.

23 Galin, D. (1974) 'Implications for psychiatry of left and right cerebral specialization', *Archives of General Psychiatry* 31: 572–583.

24 Levy, J. and Trevarthen, C. (1977) 'Perception, semantic and phonetic aspects of elementary language processes in split-brain patients', *Brain* 100: 105–118.

25 Wada, J.R. (1949) 'A new method for the determination of the side of cerebral speech dominance: a preliminary report on the intracarotid injection of sodium amytal in man', *Igaku to Seibutsugaku* 14: 221–222.

26 Deglin, V.L. (1976) 'Split brain', *The Unesco Courier* (Jan.): 5–32.

27 Blakeslee, T.R. (1980) *The Right Brain*, London: Macmillan Press.

28 Ardila, A. and Ostrosky-Solis, F. (eds) (1984) *The Right Hemisphere*, Monographs in Neuroscience, vol. 1, New York and London: Gordon & Breach Publishers.

29 Benson, F.D. and Zaidel, E. (eds) (1985) *The Dual Brain*, New York: Guilford Press.

30 Ottoson, D. (ed.) (1987) *Duality and Unity of the Brain*, Wenner-Gren International Symposium Series, vol. 47, London: Macmillan Press.
31 Geschwind, N. and Galaburda, A.M. (1987) *Cerebral Lateralization*, Cambridge, Mass.: MIT Press.
32 Wyke, B. (1960) *Proceedings*.

3 Evidence for the hypnotic state as a right hemisphere-orientated task

1 Zimbardo, P., Maslach, C. and Marshall, G. (1972) 'Hypnosis and the psychology of behavioural control', in *Hypnosis: Research Developments and Perspectives*, E. Fromm and R. Shor (eds) Chicago and New York: Aldine-Atherton.
2 Bramwell, J.M. (1921) *Hypnotism: Its History Theory and Practice*, 3rd edn, London: Rider, pp. 114–139.
3 Cutting, J. (1990) *The Right Cerebral Hemisphere and Psychiatric Disorders*, Oxford: Oxford University Press.
4 Efron, R. (1963) 'Temporal perception, aphasia, and déjà vu', *Brain* 86: 403–424.
5 Cutting, *The Right Cerebral Hemisphere*.
6 Humphrey, M.E. and Zangwill O.L. (1951) 'Cessation of dreaming after brain injury', *Journal of Neurology, Neurosurgery and Psychiatry* 14: 320–325.
7 Penfield W. and Roberts L. (1959) *Speech and Brain Mechanisms*, Princeton, NJ: Princeton University Press.
8 Greenberg, M.S. and Farah, M.J. (1986) 'The laterality of dreaming', *Brain and Cognition* 5: 307–321.
9 Cohen, David B. (1977) 'Changes in REM dream content during the night, implications for a hypothesis in cerebral dominance across REM periods', *Perceptual and Motor Skills* 44: 1267–1277.
10 Joseph, R. (1988) 'The right cerebral hemisphere: emotion, body-image, dreams, awareness', *Journal of Clinical Psychology* 42: 507–518.
11 Hogan, M. (1982) 'Effect of hypnosis on brainstem auditory evoked response', 9th International Congress of Hypnosis and Psychosomatic Medicine, Glasgow.
12 Hilgard, J.R. (1970) *Personality and Hypnosis*, Chicago: Chicago University Press.
13 Jones, G.H. and Miller, J.J. (1981) 'Functional test of the corpus callosum in schizophrenia', *British Journal of Psychiatry* 139: 553–557.
14 Sheppard, G., Manchanda, R., Gruzelier, J., Hirsch, S., Wise, R., Frackowiak, R, and Jones, T. (1983) 'O Positron Emission Tomography scanning in predominantly never-treated acute schizophrenic patients', *Lancet* (December 24/31): 1448–1452.
15 Gruzelier, J. and Hammond, N. (1976) 'A dominant hemisphere temporal lobe disorder?' Research communication in *Journal of Psychology, Psychiatry, and Behaviour* 1: 33–72.
16 Day, M.E. (1964) 'An eye movement phenomenon relating to attention, thought and anxiety', *Perceptual and Motor Skills* 19: 443–446.

17 Bakan, P. (1969) 'Hypnotisability, laterality of eye movement and functional brain asymmetry', *Perceptual and Motor Skills* 28: 927–932.
18 Gur, R.E. and Gur R.C. (1975) 'Cerebral activation as measured by subjects' lateral eye movements, influenced by experimenter location', *Neuropsychologica* 13: 35–34.
19 Erlichman H. and Weinberger, A. (1979) 'Lateral eye movements and hemispheric asymmetry', *Psychology Bulletin* 85: 1080–1101.
20 Graham, K.R. and Pernicano, K. (1979) 'Autokinetic effects under hypnosis', *American Journal of Clinical Psychology* 22: 2.
21 Frumkin, L.R., Ripley, H.S. and Cox G.B, (1978) 'Changes in cerebral lateralization with hypnosis', *Journal of Biology and Psychiatry* 13(6): 741–750.
22 Ullyett, G., Akpinar, S. and Itill, T. (1974) 'Quantitative EEG analysis during hypnosis', *American Journal of Psychiatry* 128: 799.
23 Galin, D. and Ornstein, R. (1972) 'Lateral specialization of cognitive mode: an EEG study', *Psychophysiology* 9: 412–418.
24 MacLeod-Morgan, C. and Lack, L. (1982) 'Hemispheric specificity: a physiological concomitant of hypnotizability', *Psychophysiology* 19: 687–690.
25 Mészáros, I., Bányai, E. and Greguss, A. (1982) 'Evoked potential correlates of verbal versus imagery coding in hypnosis', Paper read at 9th International Congress of Hypnosis and Psychosomatic Medicine, Glasgow.
26 Mészáros, I., Bányai, E.I. and Greguss, A. (1986) 'Enhanced right hemisphere activation during hypnosis: EEG and behavioural task performance evidence', Paper presented at the Proceedings of the 3rd International Conference of the International Organization of Psychophysiology, Vienna.
27 Crawford, H.J., Mézáros, I. and Szabó, Cs. (1989) 'EEG activation of low and high hypnotizables during waking and hypnosis; rest, math, and imaginal tasks', in *Hypnosis*, D. Waxman, D.L. Pedersen, I. Wilkie and P. Mellett, Whurr Publisher, pp. 86–91.
28 Gruzelier, J.H., Brow, T., Perry, A., Rhonder, J. and Thomas, M. (1984) 'Hypnotic susceptibility a lateral predisposition and altered cerebral asymmetry under hypnosis', *International Journal of Psychophysiology* 2: 131–139.
29 Ibid.
30 MacLeod-Morgan and Lack, 'Hemispheric specificity'.
31 Luria, A.R. and Simernitskaya, E.G. (1977) 'Interhemispheric relations and the functions of the minor hemisphere', *Neuropsychologica* 15: 175.
32 Reiff, R. and Scheerer, M. (1959) *Memory and Hypnotic Age Regression*, New York: International Universities Press.
33 Erickson, M.H. (1965) 'A special enquiry with Aldous Huxley into the nature and character of various states of consciousness', *American Journal of Clinical Hypnosis* 8: 17.
34 Freud, S. and Breuer, J. (1895) *Studien über Hysterie*, Vienna.
35 Hilgard, E.R. and Hilgard, J.R. (1989) *Hypnosis and the Relief of Pain*, Kaufman Inc., pp. 166–169.

36 Gazzaniga, M.S. (1972) 'One brain – two minds', *American Scientist* 60: 311–312.
37 Frumkin, L.R., Ripley, H.S. and Cox, G.B. (1978) 'Changes in cerebral lateralization with hypnosis', *Journal of Biological Psychiatry* 13(6): 741–750.
38 Orne, M.T. (1951) 'The mechanisms of hypnotic age-regression', *Journal of Abnormal Psychology*, Monographs 76 (3, Pt.2): 56.
39 Zaidel, E. (1985) 'Callosal dynamics and right hemisphere language', *Neurology and Neurobiology* 17: 435–439.
40 Bogen, J.E. (1987) 'Partial hemispheric independence with the neo-commissures intact', in *Brain Circuits and Functions of the Mind*, Cambridge: Cambridge University Press.
41 Ottoson, D. (1986) *Duality and Unity of the Brain*, London: Macmillan Press.
42 Sperry, R.W. (1968) 'Hemispheric deconnection and unity in conscious awareness', *American Psychologist* 23: 723–733.
43 Levy, J., Trevarthen, C. and Sperry, R.W. (1972) 'Perception of bilateral chimeric figures following hemispheric deconnection', *Brain* 95: 61–78.
44 Levy, J. (1970) 'Information processing in the disconnected hemispheres', Unpublished thesis, California Institute of Technology.

4 Cameral analysis

1 Levy, J. and Trevarthen, C. (1977) 'Perceptual, semantic and phonetic aspects of language processes in split-brain patients', *Brain* 100: 105–118.
2 Gazzaniga, M.S. (1972) 'One brain – two minds', *American Scientist* 60: 311.2.
3 Monrad-Krohn, G.H. (1947) 'The prosodic qualities of speech and its disorders', *Acta Psychologica et Neurologica Scandinavica* 22: 255–269.
4 Weintraub, S., Mesulam, M. and Kramer, L. (1981) 'Disturbances in prosody: a right-hemisphere contribution to language', *Archives Neurology* 38 (December): 742–744.
5 Shepherd, M. *Sherlock Holmes and the Case of Dr. Freud*, London: Tavistock Publications.
6 Gellner, E. *The Psychoanalytic Movement*, London: Paladin Press.
7 Tyler, P. (1991) 'Introduction', *British Journal of Psychiatry* 159, Supplement, 12: 5.
8 Gray, J.A. (1982) *The Neuropsychology of Anxiety*, Oxford: Clarendon Press.
9 Eccles, J.C. (1969) 'The inhibitory pathways of the central nervous system', Sherrington Lectures IX, Liverpool University Press.
10 Aserinsky, E. and Kleitman, N. (1953) 'Regular occurring periods of eye motility and concomitant phenomena during sleep', *Science* 118: 273–274.
11 Dement, W.C. and Kleitman, N. (1957) 'The relation of eye move-

ments during sleep to dream activity; an objective method for the study of dreaming', *Journal of Experimental Psychology* 53: 339–346.

12 Hernandez-Peon, R. (1967) 'Neurophysiology, phylogeny, and functional significance of dreaming', *Experimental Neurology* 4: 106–125.

13 Cohen, D. (1979) *Sleep and Dreaming*, International Series in Experimental Psychology, H.J. Eysenck (ed.) vol. 23, Oxford: Pergamon Press.

14 Crisp, A.H., Kame, J., Potamianos, G. and Bhat, A.V. (1985) 'Cerebral hemisphere function and laterality of migraine', *Psychotherapy Psychosomatics* 43: 49–55.

15 Crisp, A.H., Levett, G., Davies, P., Rose, F.C. and Coltheart, M. (1989) 'Cerebral hemisphere function and migraine', *Journal of Psychiatric Research* 23 (3/4): 201–212.

5   Abreaction

1 Freud, S. and Breuer, J. (1895) 'Studien über Hysterie', quoted in *An Autobiographical Study*, 1936, Freud, S., The International Psycho-Analytical Library, No. 26., pp. 37–38.

2 Ibid., pp. 38–39.

3 Brown, W. (1938) *Psychological Methods of Healing*, London: University of London Press, p. 20.

4 Culpin, M. (1920) *Psychoneuroses of War and Peace*, London: Cambridge University Press, p. 16.

5 Brown, *Psychological Methods of Healing*.

6 Ibid.

7 Horsley, J. S. (1936) 'Narco-analysis: a new technique in short-cut psychotherapy; a comparison with other methods', *Lancet* 1: 55.

8 Gray, J. A. (1982) *The Neuropsychology of Anxiety*, Oxford: Clarendon Press, pp. 300–301.

9 Wyke, B. (1960) 'Neurological mechanisms in hypnosis; some recent advances in the study of hypnotic phenomena', *Proceedings of the Dental and Medical Society for the Study of Hypnosis* (March), p. 21.

10 Gray, *The Neuropsychology of Anxiety*.

11 Sargant, W. and Slater, E. (1940) 'Amnesic syndromes in war', *Lancet* 2: 1

12 Shorvon, H. J. and Sargant, W. (1947) 'Excitatory abreaction: with special reference to its mechanism and the use of ether', *Journal of Mental Science* 393 (Oct.) 709–732.

13 Sargant, W. and Shorvon, H. J. (1945) 'Acute war neurosis: with special reference to Pavlov's experimental observations and the mechanisms of abreaction', *Archives of Neurology and Psychiatry* 545 (Oct.): 231–240.

6   Cameral analysis and art form

1 Lewis-Williams, J.D. and Dowson, T.A. (1988) 'The signs of all times – entoptic phenomena in Upper Paleolithic art', *Current Anthropology* 29 (2) (April): 201–245.

2 Oliver, L. (1989) 'The use of hypnosis as a therapeutic technique by traditional African healers', in *Hypnosis, 4th European Congress at Oxford*, D. Waxman, D.L. Pedersen, I. Wilkie, and P. Mellett, (eds) London and N.J.: Whurr Publisher

7   Cameral analysis and music and dance

1 Bradshaw, J.L. and Nettleton, N.C. (1983) *Cerebral Hemisphere Asymmetry*, Englewood Cliffs, NJ: Prentice-Hall.
2 Gates, A. and Bradshaw, J.L. (1977) 'The role of the hemispheres in music', *Brain and Language* 4: 403–431.
3 Gordon, H.W. (1983) 'Music and the right hemisphere', in Andrew Young (ed.), *Functions of the Right Hemisphere*, London; Academic Press, pp. 65–86.
4 Bradshaw and Nettleton, *Cerebral Hemisphere Asymmetry*.
5 Gates and Bradshaw, 'The role of the hemispheres in music'.
6 Bever, T.G. and Chiarello, R.J. (1974) 'Cerebral dominance in musicians and non-musicians', *Science* 185: 127–139.
7 Shipkowcnsky, N. (1977) 'Musical therapy in the field of psychiatry and neurology', in *Music and the Brain* M. Critchely and R.A. Henson (eds) London: Heinemann, pp. 433–455.
8 Radin, P. (1948) 'Music and medicine among primitive peoples', in *Music and Medicine*, D.M. Schullian and M. Schoen (eds) New York: Schuman, pp. 3–24.
9 Densmore, F.R. (1948) 'The use of music in the treatment of the sick', in *Music and Medicine*, D.M. Schullian and M. Schoen (eds) New York: Schuman, pp. 25–46.
10 Meinecke, B., (1948) 'Music and medicine in classical antiquity', in *Music and Medicine*, D.M. Schullian and M. Schoen (eds) New York: Schuman, pp. 47–95.
11 Ellenberger, H.F. (1974) 'Psychiatry from ancient to modern times', in *American Handbook of Psychiatry*, Silvano Arieti (ed.) 2nd edn, New York: Basic Books, pp. 3–27.
12 Akstein, D. (1987) 'Reizuber flutung als Therapieform: die Terpsichoretrancetherapie (TTT)' in *Ethnopsychotherapie*, A. Dittrich and C. Sharfetter (eds), Stuttgart: Ferdinand Enke Verlag.
13 Akstein, D. (1992) *Un Voyage à travers la transe – la terpischore transethérapie*, Paris: Ed. Tchou.
14 Sargant, W. and Fraser R. (1938) 'Inducing light hypnosis by hyperventilation', *Lancet* II: 778.
15 Editorial, *Journal of the Royal Society of Medicine* 74 (Jan. 1981): 1–4.
16 Wyke, B. (1960) *Proceedings of the Dental and Medical Society for the Study of Hypnosis* (March): 21.
17 Lum, L.C. (1987) 'Hyperventilation syndromes in medicine and psychiatry: a review', *Journal of the Royal Society of Medicine* 80 (April): 229–231.
18 Lum, 'Hyperventilation syndromes'.
19 Gruzelier, J.H., Brow, T., Perry, A., Rhonder, J. and Thomas, M.

(1984) 'Hypnotic susceptibility', *International Journal of Psychophysiology* 2: 131–139.
20 Gates and Bradshaw, 'The role of the hemispheres in music'.

8 Cameral analysis and poetry

1 Ricks, C.B. (1987) *The Force of Poetry*, Oxford: Oxford University Press.
2 Ibid.
3 Cox, M. and Theilgaard, A. (1987) *Mutative Metaphors in Psychotherapy*, London: Tavistock Publications.
4 Bachelard, G. (1969) *The Poetics of Space*, Boston: Beacon Press.

9 Multiple personality syndrome

1 Völgyesi, F.A. (1966) *Hypnosis of Man and Animals*, M.W. Hamilton, trans., London: Baillière, Tindall, Cassell.
2 Paracelsus, P.A. (1646) *Opera*, vol. 2, Strasbourg.
3 Plumer, W.S. (1859–1860) 'Mary Reynolds: a case of double consciousness', *Harper's New Monthly Magazine* XX: 807–812.
4 Myers, F.W. (1886) 'Multiplex personality', *The Nineteenth Century* (Nov.): 648–666.
5 Gott, P.S., Hughes, E. and Whipple, K. (1984) 'Voluntary control of two lateralized conscious states: validation by electrical and behavioural studies', *Neuropsychologia* 22(1): 65–72.
6 Milgram, S. (1963) 'Behavioural study of obedience', *Journal of Abnormal and Social Psychology* 67: 371–378.
7 Milgram, S. (1974) *Obedience to Authority*, London: Harper & Row.
8 Shatzman, M. (1980) *The Story of Ruth*, London: Gerald Duckworth & Co.
9 Bliss, E.L. (1986) *Multiple Personality, Allied Disorders and Hypnosis*, Oxford: Oxford University Press.

Index